The Practice Paradox

Avoid Burnout. Embrace Balance.
Build the Practice of Your Dreams.

By: Luke Infinger and
Dr. Kyle Fagala

THE PRACTICE PARADOX

Copyright © 2025 Luke Infinger and Dr. Kyle Fagala

Published by: Expert Author Press
https://www.expertauthorpress.com/

ISBN-13: 978-1-990476-18-1

Canadian Address:
767 Eastvale Dr.
Ottawa, Ontario, Canada K1J 6Z9
Phone: (604) 941-3041
info@expertauthorpress.com

Contents

Section VI: Purpose & Reflection

Preface

"We always hope for the easy fix: the one simple change that will erase a problem in a stroke. But few things in life work this way. Instead, success requires making a hundred small steps go right - one after the other, no slip ups, no goofs, everyone pitching in." — Atul Gawande

This book was born from two journeys that ran in parallel, eventually converging around a shared realization: success in orthodontics often comes at a hidden cost.

Dr. Kyle Fagala: Growing up in Jonesboro, Arkansas, with a scientist for a father and an English teacher for a mother, I learned early that life's most rewarding pursuits require both precision and passion. Still, I never imagined that years after completing my orthodontic residency at the University of Tennessee with dreams of building my ideal practice, I'd one day be writing about work-life balance rather than bracket systems or wire sequences (although, we do discuss some of that in chapter 9).

Luke Infinger: Similarly, I never expected my journey from motion graphics at SCAD to co-founding HIP Creative would lead me to help orthodontists and dentists escape the very trap I had fled when I left New York City for a more balanced and prosperous life in Pensacola, FL. Yet here we are, addressing what might be the most important issue in private practice that no one is talking about: the silent epidemic of burnout among the very professionals dedicated to creating beautiful smiles, joy, confidence, and happiness.

We came together around a simple but profound truth: the way most orthodontists are trained to succeed sets them up for paradox. They achieve professional milestones but often at the expense of personal fulfillment. We knew there had to be a better way.

This book is our answer to that realization. It's not another management manual or quick-fix playbook. It's an invitation to rethink what it means to succeed in practice and in life, and to see that the two are not opposites. Our goal is to show you how to reclaim joy, integrate purpose, and build systems that support, not consume your life.

We are deeply grateful to our families, who lived this journey with us; to our colleagues and mentors, who modeled both the challenges and possibilities of this profession; and to the many doctors who opened up about their struggles and triumphs, reminding us that no one is truly alone in facing the paradox.

This preface is a doorway into the spirit of the book: honest, personal, and rooted in lived experience. In the pages ahead, you'll find not only strategies and frameworks, but stories and insights that can help you create a life and practice that feel whole.

Thank you for picking up this book. We hope it encourages, challenges, and supports you as you chart your own path forward.

Introduction: Entering the Practice Paradox

It was Sunday evening, and Dr. James sat at the dinner table with his family, but his mind was already at the office. His daughter was telling him about her soccer game, but he barely heard her words. He was running through tomorrow's schedule in his head. When his son spilled a glass of water, James snapped, the frustration spilling out sharper than he intended. His wife gave him a look across the table, one that carried both weariness and disappointment. He tried to pull himself back into the moment, but the knot in his stomach only tightened. The weekend had been no refuge. Half of Saturday had been lost to catching up on lab cases, and Sunday afternoon, he had ducked away to check emails while his kids played outside.

This wasn't the life he imagined when he dreamed of becoming an orthodontist. He had wanted to help people, to give them confidence, to create a better life for his family. But now, as he pushed food around his plate, all he could feel was dread for Monday morning. The practice that had once felt like a calling had become the source of his tension, straining his marriage, stealing his presence with his children, and leaving him unwell in body and spirit.

Dentistry and orthodontics were never meant to feel this way. What begins as a noble calling too often becomes a grind. Across the profession, burnout has become the silent epidemic. On paper, practices look prosperous: patient loads are steady, reputations strong, and financials healthy. Yet behind those numbers, the people running them often feel drained, disconnected, and quietly unfulfilled.

This is the paradox we're here to name. It's the cultural myth that professional success can only be earned through relentless sacrifice. That the only path to excellence is giving everything, all the time, until there is nothing left. The result is predictable—strained marriages, missed family milestones, physical exhaustion, and practices that consume the very people who built them.

We believe the profession has reached a turning point. Rates of stress, depression, and disengagement are rising. The pandemic only amplified what was already there: cracks in the culture of dentistry that too many have learned to ignore. Doctors who seemed to be thriving began to share, quietly and sometimes reluctantly, that the cost of their "success" was unsustainable.

Through our work with hundreds of dentists and orthodontists, helping them scale, grow, and strengthen their marketing and operations, we discovered something crucial. Growth alone is not the key to success. The deeper foundation lies in fulfillment and in designing a practice that supports the life you want to live, the meaning you want to experience, and the impact you want to make in the world. We realized that we could not, in good conscience, continue to help practices expand and become "more successful" without addressing this critical factor.

That realization is what shaped this book. In the chapters ahead, you'll discover how fulfillment, purpose, and alignment transform not only practices but also lives. We've seen it firsthand: when doctors align their practices with who they are and the lives they want to live, the result is joy, clarity, and energy. This alignment doesn't just improve the bottom line; it restores the calling that brought you into this profession in the first place.

This is not another practice management manual or a checklist of quick fixes. What you'll find here is a guide for integrating professional success with personal well-being, rooted in lived experience and tested through real practices.

This book is for you if your practice is thriving but you feel hollow inside. If you dread Sunday nights even though your numbers look strong. If you want to be excellent at your craft while still living fully with your family, your friends, and yourself. It takes courage to face these truths, but that courage is the first step toward freedom.

Our promise is simple: the paradox can end. In these pages, you'll discover a roadmap to reclaim joy, redefine success, and build a practice that supports your life rather than consumes it. And so we begin, fittingly, with **Chapter One: Happiness vs. Joy**, because that is where fulfillment truly starts.

What to Expect from this Book:

The Practice Paradox is organized into six sections that reflect the journey of building a practice—and a life—that is both successful and sustainable. Each section focuses on a key domain of fulfillment, moving from internal alignment to external execution.

I. Foundations of Fulfillment

II. Communication & Connection

III. Identity & Leadership

IV. Practice Growth & Operations

V. Life Beyond the Clinic

VI. Purpose & Reflection

Section I: Foundations of Fulfillment

Discover:

Chapter 1 – Happiness vs. Joy: Why joy, not fleeting happiness, is the true foundation of fulfillment in your practice and life.

Chapter 1: Happiness vs. Joy

By: Dr. Kyle Fagala

The Silent Sacrifice:
When Your Dream Practice Becomes Your Prison

Dr. Sarah hadn't seen her daughter's bedtime routine in three weeks.

The practice was thriving—revenue up 23%, patient satisfaction scores excellent—yet she sat in her car every evening wondering how success could feel so much like failure.

Sound familiar?

You've built the practice others envy—bustling schedule, excellent clinical outcomes, healthy revenue—yet something feels fundamentally off. The success that should taste sweet has become strangely hollow.

You're not alone.

The very practice Sarah had dreamed of building now felt like it was running her life instead of fueling it. This is the central paradox of modern practice: the traits that make you successful —discipline, perfectionism, and relentless drive —can also become the very things that burn you out. The solution isn't abandoning your ambition. It's building a practice that aligns with your values and fuels your joy.

This first chapter is about reclaiming your foundation and introduces the framework that will guide the rest of the book. The J.O.Y. Framework is the antidote to burnout and the path to reclaiming the life you actually want. Before we talk about systems, marketing, or growth, we must first answer: What does joy in practice look like for you? When your daily decisions are aligned with your values and anchored in purpose, your practice becomes a source of energy rather than exhaustion.

The Mental Health Crisis Nobody Talks About

The numbers paint a sobering picture of our profession's hidden struggle.

Depression rates have surged dramatically across the United States, with lifetime diagnosis rates jumping nearly 10 percentage points from 2015 to 2023 alone (Gallup, 2023). Among dental professionals, the crisis runs even deeper. Recent studies show that 44% of dentists experience burnout symptoms—a rate that significantly exceeds most other professions (BDJ Open, 2024).

Consider these stark realities:

Suicide rates among dental professionals rank among the highest of any healthcare field (University of Melbourne, 2023)

Heart disease and emotional illness plague our colleagues at alarming rates (Dr. Randy Lang, "Stress in Dentistry - It Could Kill You!" Oral Health Group, 2017)

The very tools meant to connect us have become sources of chronic stress and distraction

Every day, talented dentists and orthodontists wake up to a troubling reality: **the practice they've poured their lives into has become a source of exhaustion rather than fulfillment.**

We've been conditioned to believe that sacrifice is the necessary price of excellence—that we must choose between being outstanding clinicians or present parents, engaged community members, and whole human beings.

This false dichotomy forms the core of what we call **"The Practice Paradox"**—the misguided belief that professional success and personal fulfillment exist in opposition to one another.

But here's the paradox within the paradox:

In some of the world's poorest regions, researchers observe profound joy and contentment among people facing material hardships we can barely imagine. Meanwhile, in our comfortable offices with state-of-the-art equipment and six-figure incomes, many clinicians struggle with emptiness and despair.

It's clear this isn't about money or circumstances—it's about something deeper.

What If There's Another Way?

What if the traditional model of practice management—with its all-consuming demands and endless sacrifice—isn't the only path forward?

The journey toward a more balanced practice life begins with understanding a fundamental distinction that most of us have never been taught to make: **the crucial difference between happiness and joy.** It's the foundation upon which sustainable success is built.

The promise of this book isn't merely a less stressful workday—though that will certainly come. **The real promise is reclaiming your vision of what practicing dentistry or orthodontics was meant to be: a profession that enhances your life rather than consumes it.**

Your practice should serve your life, not the other way around.

The Weight of a White Coat

Dr. Michael pulled into his reserved parking space at 7:15 PM. The office had closed at 5:00, but he stayed to catch up on patient files. The dashboard clock glowed in the growing darkness. He shut off the engine and sat still, listening to the cooling tick of the motor.

He thought about calling Rhea. He had missed dinner again. Their anniversary dinner. Twenty years of marriage compressed into a text message apology and a promise to make it up to her this weekend. Michael knew the promise rang hollow.

The steering wheel felt cool under his palms. He remembered the day he had bought this car—a reward after paying off his dental school loans. That had been eight years ago, and he had barely enjoyed it. The leather seats had aged better than he had. Michael caught his reflection in the rearview mirror. The lines around his eyes had deepened. His father had those same lines, but his had come with laughter. Michael's came from peering into countless mouths under operatory lights, shoulders hunched over patients in chairs that never seemed positioned quite right.

His phone buzzed. A text from Dr. Winters, his mentor from dental school: "Still on for golf tomorrow?" Michael had forgotten. He typed "Can't make it" then deleted it. He remembered Winters' advice from years ago: "A dental practice should give you freedom, not take it away." Michael had nodded then, not understanding. Now he understood too well.

The Happiness Trap That's Killing Your Joy

There's more than a semantic difference between "happiness" and "joy," and that difference is foundational to how we experience our professional lives.

Happiness often comes as a fleeting response to external circumstances: completing a difficult procedure, receiving a positive patient review, or hitting a revenue milestone. It arrives quickly and departs just as fast, leaving us constantly chasing the next achievement.

Joy, by contrast, emerges from alignment between our daily actions and our deepest values. It's the orthodontist who builds a practice allowing them to do exceptional work while still attending their children's soccer games. It's the satisfaction that comes not from isolated wins but from knowing your professional journey reflects who you truly are.

Research tracking dental school graduates over their first decade reveals a sobering truth: **income and practice size show little correlation with reported life satisfaction, while factors like work-life balance, sense of purpose, and alignment with personal values are the strongest predictors of long-term career fulfillment.**

The constant pursuit of happiness through achievements, acquisitions, and accolades leaves many clinicians trapped on what psychologists call the "hedonic treadmill"—running faster but never actually advancing.

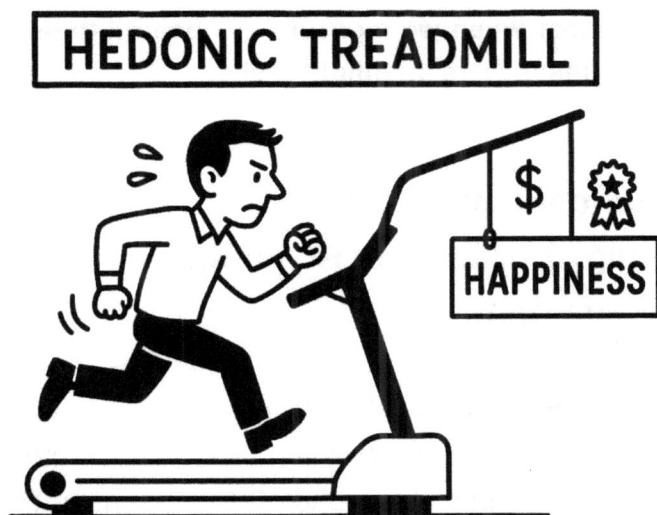

HEDONIC TREADMILL

$

HAPPINESS

Your Brain Is Working Against You

Our brains are wired for the quick hit of happiness. Evolution favored immediate rewards because they helped our ancestors survive. But in the modern context of building a sustainable practice, this biological tendency works against us, pushing us toward choices that feel good now but damage our long-term well-being.

The comparison trap amplifies this problem. We see colleagues' success without the full context of their struggles. Posts about latest cases, new equipment, and practice milestones create immediate pressure to match or exceed their achievements, regardless of whether those achievements align with our own values.

"Comparison is the thief of joy" is a truth that becomes painfully clear when we measure our behind-the-scenes reality against others' highlight reels.

The Fundamental Shift: Creating Your Life vs. Reacting to Circumstances

This shift requires what author T. Harv Eker calls proactive living—the recognition that you create your life rather than simply responding to circumstances. In his book *Secrets of the Millionaire Mind*, Eker identifies this as the fundamental difference: instead of believing "life happens to me," joy-centered clinicians adopt the mindset **"I create my life."**

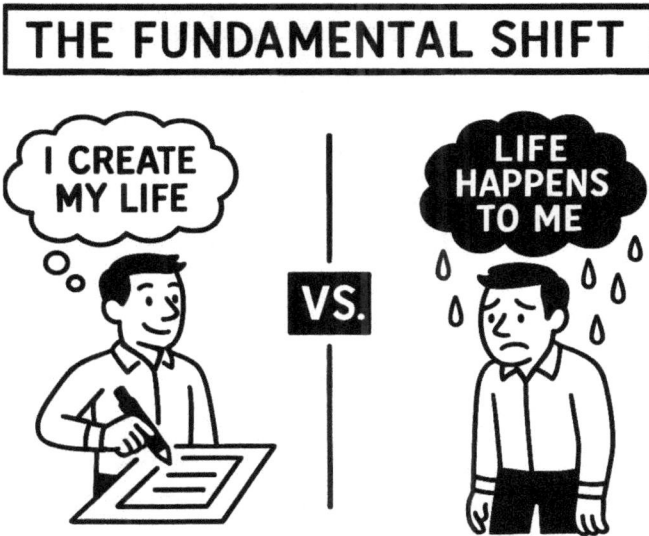

Joy requires patience and intentionality. It emerges when we craft our professional lives around purpose rather than pleasure alone. Building a joyful practice means sometimes saying no to opportunities that might bring short-term happiness but don't align with your ultimate vision.

It means measuring success not just by production numbers but by how well your practice enables the life you want to live.

Through our marketing agency work and connections with hundreds of orthodontists and dentists, we've observed a consistent pattern: those who prioritize joy over mere happiness build more sustainable practices and experience greater personal fulfillment. They create practices that others want to be part of. Patients sense the authenticity, and team members are drawn to leaders who embody purpose rather than just pursuing profit.

The Science of Delayed Gratification

The marshmallow experiment remains one of psychology's most famous studies. Stanford researcher Walter Mischel offered children a choice: eat one marshmallow immediately or wait fifteen minutes and receive two. Those who delayed gratification showed better life outcomes decades later, including higher SAT scores, lower BMI, and greater career success.

This principle applies powerfully to dental practice management.

Every day, clinicians face choices between immediate gratification and long-term success. The choices that build sustainable practices rarely deliver instant rewards.

Neuroscience helps explain why these choices feel so difficult. When faced with immediate rewards, our limbic system activates strongly. The prefrontal cortex must work overtime to override these impulses. It's like having two competing operating systems: one ancient and focused on immediate survival, one evolved and capable of long-term planning.

Think of your practice as a garden rather than a vending machine.

Vending machines provide instant results—insert money, receive product. Gardens require consistent attention over time before yielding their harvest. The most successful clinicians approach their careers with a gardener's patience.

Research published in the *Journal of the American Dental Association* found that clinicians who maintained three to six months of operating expenses in liquid reserves reported 43% lower stress levels during economic downturns compared to those operating with minimal cash reserves.

Neurochemistry supports this: when we successfully resist immediate temptation for future benefit, our brains release both dopamine and serotonin, creating deeper, more sustainable satisfaction than quick dopamine hits.

The paradox of practice growth is that the actions most likely to produce sustainable success often feel uncomfortable in the moment.

Investing in continuing education when production numbers are tight. Limiting your schedule to maintain quality rather than packing in more starts. Taking time away from the practice for personal renewal when the schedule is full.

What would your practice look like if every decision considered not just tomorrow's production report but the quality of your life five years from now?

The Value-Vision Decision Framework

Making decisions that align with your personal values and long-term vision isn't just good philosophy—**it's good business.**

When clinicians make choices that honor their core values, they experience less internal conflict, greater consistency in leadership, and stronger patient relationships.

The disconnect often begins during professional training, where clinical excellence takes center stage while clarifying personal values receives little attention. We learn to diagnose conditions and perform procedures with precision, but rarely examine how our practice model should reflect who we are as individuals.

The most fulfilled clinicians are those whose daily decisions consistently reflect their core values, not the ones who have eliminated all their problems.

Research from organizational psychology shows that professionals who reported high alignment between personal values and daily work decisions were 62% less likely to experience burnout symptoms, regardless of work hours or compensation level.

Consider the clinician who values family connection above all else but builds a practice requiring sixty-hour work weeks—the dissonance creates psychological strain that no amount of financial success can resolve.

The traditional practice management model often presents a false choice: sacrifice your personal values for professional success, or accept mediocrity to maintain work-life balance. This either-or thinking misses the more powerful third option: designing a practice that serves both your professional ambitions and personal values simultaneously.

The shift from reactive to values-based decision making requires developing "pause power"—the ability to create space between stimulus and response. Values-aligned clinicians ask different questions: "Does this opportunity align with who I want to be and where I want my practice to go?" "Will this decision enhance or compromise the life I'm trying to build?"

The J.O.Y. Decision Framework

The J.O.Y. Decision Framework offers a structured approach to making choices that generate sustainable fulfillment in professional practice. This evidence-based model synthesizes insights from positive psychology, organizational behavior, and years of research culminating in my "Embrace Happiness" lecture, where I identified the **Ten Foundations of Joy**—the key habits and patterns among clinicians who successfully cultivate lasting joy in their careers.

Through extensive conversations with colleagues and analysis of what distinguishes fulfilled clinicians from those trapped in the Practice Paradox, I've distilled these findings into a systematic framework: **Journey, Outcomes, You**—three interconnected dimensions that transform how we evaluate and make decisions.

The J.O.Y. Framework Architecture

I. **J – Journey – The Process Dimension** – Focuses on your daily practices and processes—how you approach each day, each patient interaction, and each decision with intentionality rather than reactivity.

II. **O – Outcomes – The Results Dimension** – Emphasizes what you're actually creating and prioritizing—the relationships, experiences, and contributions that provide lasting meaning beyond production metrics.

III. **Y – You – The Personal Dimension** – Establishes your personal capacity—understanding who you are, maintaining your health, and building the self-awareness necessary for authentic decision-making.

J.O.Y. DECISION FRAMEWORK

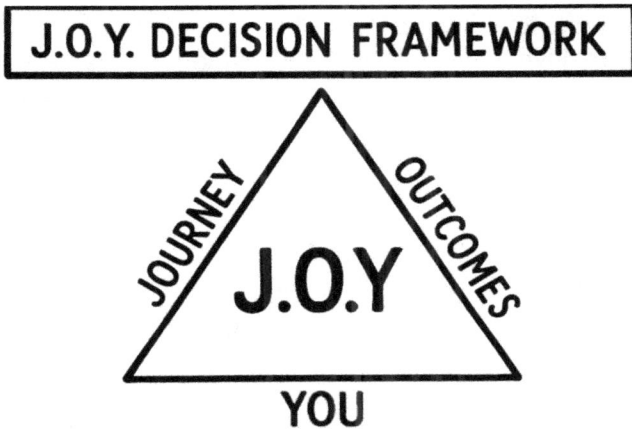

J = JOURNEY focuses on your daily practices and processes

O = OUTCOMES emphasizes what you're actually creating and prioritizing

Y = YOU establishes your personal foundation

<u>Journey</u>: The Process Dimension

Your daily journey determines whether you experience fulfillment or frustration. The most joyful clinicians have mastered four key process elements:

1. **Live in the Now** - Being fully present during patient interactions rather than mentally planning the next case or worrying about production numbers. Present-moment awareness reduces stress and improves both clinical outcomes and patient satisfaction.

2. **Be Humble & Grateful** - Regular gratitude practice that rewires attention toward what's working rather

than exclusively focusing on problems. This isn't positive thinking but strategic attention management—gratitude literally changes what your brain notices.

3. **Get Organized & Be Intentional** - Applying systems like the Eisenhower Matrix to distinguish between urgent and important activities, to make sure long-term priorities don't get crowded out by daily pressures.

4. **Stop the Comparisons** - Breaking free from the comparison trap and replacing it with celebration of others' success. This requires conscious practice when others' highlight reels constantly compete for our attention.

<u>Outcomes</u>: The Results Dimension

This dimension focuses on what you're actually creating through your practice—results that provide lasting meaning beyond financial metrics:

5. **Experiences > Things** - Prioritizing investments that create memories and relationships over material accumulation. Research consistently shows that experiential purchases provide more lasting satisfaction than material ones.

6. **Give Back** - Finding ways to serve beyond your practice, whether through missions or community programs (like Mid-South Mission of Mercy in Saddle Creek Orthodontics' case, or Embrace Memphis, our

nonprofit supporting families in adoption and foster care). Service creates what psychologists call "eudaimonic well-being"—satisfaction from meaning and purpose rather than pleasure alone.

<u>You</u>: The Personal Dimension

Your personal foundation determines your capacity for both intentional journey practices and meaningful outcomes:

7. **Understand, Love, and Accept Yourself** - Using validated tools like Myers-Briggs or StrengthsFinder to recognize your natural patterns and work with them rather than against them.

8. **Work on Your Mindset** - Developing T. Harv Eker's "I create my life" mentality rather than the reactive "life happens to me" approach.

9. **Exercise, Diet, and Sleep** - Maintaining physical health as the foundation for mental clarity and emotional resilience.

10. **Seek Professional Help** - Normalizing therapy, counseling, and expert consultation. The most successful clinicians view seeking help as a strength and invest in their mental health as deliberately as they do their clinical skills.

Integrated Decision-Making Process

When facing choices about practice direction, scheduling, hiring, or investment, run each option through all three dimensions:

> **Journey Assessment:** How will this choice affect my ability to be present and intentional in my daily work?

> **Outcomes Evaluation:** What kind of relationships, experiences, and service opportunities does this create or eliminate?

> **You Filter:** Does this decision align with my natural strengths and values? Will this support or undermine my physical and mental health?

Research from Harvard Business School shows that leaders who score highly across multiple well-being dimensions demonstrate 79% better decision-making consistency and 65% higher long-term career satisfaction.

When you consistently make decisions that honor all three dimensions—your Journey, your desired Outcomes, and You as a person—you create what psychologists call "flourishing": a state where professional success enhances rather than compromises personal fulfillment.

The Compound Effect of Aligned Decisions

Through my research for the "Embrace Happiness" lecture and our marketing agency work with hundreds of orthodontists and dentists, I've observed a consistent pattern: **small, values-aligned decisions compound over time to create dramatically different outcomes.**

As well as providing better care, the orthodontist who consistently chooses to be fully present during patient interactions builds deeper relationships that generate more referrals and higher satisfaction. Similarly, the clinician who regularly invests in experiences over material acquisitions develops a richer perspective that makes them more innovative and resilient.

The fundamental insight is this: joy isn't a destination you reach after achieving enough success. Joy is the quality of attention and intention you bring to the journey itself.

Your Next Move

Dr. Michael, sitting in his car at 7:15 PM, represents countless clinicians caught between two worlds: the success they've achieved and the life they actually want to live. His story illustrates the Practice Paradox at its core—the misguided belief that professional excellence and personal fulfillment exist in opposition to one another.

The breakthrough comes when you realize that **sustainable success requires integration, not sacrifice.**

The most fulfilled clinicians have learned to make decisions that honor their Journey, create meaningful Outcomes, and serve You as a whole person simultaneously.

This integration requires the same discipline and intentionality you bring to clinical excellence. Just as you wouldn't perform a complex procedure without proper preparation, building a joyful practice demands structured thinking and consistent application of proven principles.

Key Takeaways

- The Practice Paradox, the belief that professional success and personal fulfillment are mutually exclusive, is a false assumption that traps many clinicians in burnout.

- Joy is a deeper, more sustainable state than happiness that's tied to purpose, not just circumstances.

- Shifting from reaction to creation in your life and work is essential to breaking free from The Practice Paradox.

- The J.O.Y. Decision Framework can help align daily choices with long-term fulfillment.

Next Steps

You don't have to master the complete system to begin experiencing change. Starting this week, you can:

Apply the J.O.Y. Framework to one significant decision - Run it through all three dimensions: How does this serve my Journey practices? What Outcomes will this create? Does this honor You as a person?

Implement a weekly 15-minute review - Reflect on your decisions through the lens of your values and long-term vision.

Choose one of the ten foundations to strengthen - Rather than trying to transform everything at once, focus on developing one element consistently for the next 30 days.

The Choice Is Yours

Dr. Michael made his choice that evening, texting Dr. Winters about golf and calling Rhea about Sedona. Those declarations of a different way of living and practicing proved to be small choices that signaled a fundamental shift from reactive survival to proactive creation of the life and practice he actually wanted.

What choice will you make?

The practice that consumes your life is waiting for tomorrow's crisis. The practice that serves your life is waiting for your next decision.

The time for integration is now. Your journey toward sustainable joy begins with the very next choice you make.

Defining joy is only the beginning. Once you've clarified what you're working toward, the first step in building alignment is communication. Your vision can't live only in your head—it has to be shared. Your team can't help you create the practice you want if they don't understand what that vision is or how to support it. Patients can't trust your care if they don't feel heard and understood.

That's why communication is the essential foundation of everything that follows. In the next chapter, we'll explore how masterful communication creates clarity, trust, and freedom in your practice—and why it's the single most important skill to build once you've defined your version of joy.

Section II: Communication & Connection

Discover:

Chapter 2 – Masterful Communication: How communication sets the stage for clarity, trust, and alignment with your team and patients.

Chapter 3 – Building Meaningful Relationships: Why investing in deeper connections with patients, colleagues, and mentors creates lasting fulfillment and success.

Chapter 2: Masterful Communication

By: Luke Infinger

Dr. Nicole would tense up whenever she overheard her staff talking to patients. The words were never wrong, exactly, but they weren't how she would've said it. Every phrase left her wishing she'd jumped in, convinced she could've handled it better. Sound familiar?

Breaking free from the Practice Paradox begins with joy. Choosing alignment with your values instead of sacrificing fulfillment for success. But joy can't stay an abstract idea. It has to show up in how you lead, how your team operates, and how your patients experience your practice.

You don't need to carry every decision in your practice alone. The real key to growth isn't more effort; it's communication. Masterful communication is what transforms your vision into reality, turning a group of employees into an empowered team and anxious patients into loyal advocates.

Words Create Worlds: Communication as Your Practice Superpower

Let's start with a hard truth: If every decision in your practice has to run through you, you've either hired the wrong people, trained them poorly, or failed to develop leaders.

Maybe all three.

That might sting, but it explains why so many practices plateau—or worse, turn into prisons. When everything depends on you, your practice can't grow. You become the bottleneck, not the engine.

Most doctors don't think of this as a communication problem. But it is.

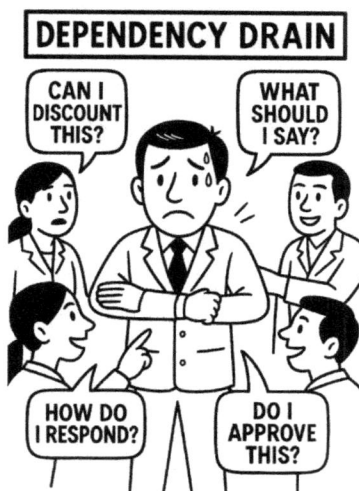

DEPENDENCY DRAIN

CAN I DISCOUNT THIS?

WHAT SHOULD I SAY?

HOW DO I RESPOND?

DO I APPROVE THIS?

Communication isn't just about clarity—it's about relationships. And strong relationships are what unlock trust. Trust gives people permission to own their roles. To act without asking. To lead without waiting for approval. And when that happens, your team starts mastering their domain. Not because you micromanaged them, but because you showed them what great leadership looks like.

This doesn't mean you check out. Great leaders stay close enough to guide but far enough to let their team grow. They build people, not dependencies. Masterful communication becomes the force multiplier—driving faster decisions, fewer conflicts, greater initiative, and better results. Done right, it's one of the rare tools that gives you something priceless back: your time, your freedom, and your life.

When communication systems falter, clinicians find themselves trapped in an endless cycle of clarification, repetition, and damage control. You've likely experienced days where you're constantly pulled into conversations that your team could have handled, leaving you exhausted and your staff dependent. In turn, this dependency creates a long-term lag that becomes unsustainable for both practice growth and personal wellbeing.

The breakthrough comes when you realize communication is not just about what you say. It is about creating systems that speak clearly even when you are not in the room. The key is equipping your team with simple, repeatable frameworks and the right tools to support them. This makes communication scalable across your practice. You stop being the message and start designing the system that delivers it.

But systems alone aren't enough.

You can have SOPs, templates, scripts, and dashboards— but if the mood is sour, the trust is gone, or the culture is toxic, no one follows the playbook. At best, they go through the motions. At worst, they ignore it entirely.

Here's the deeper truth:

Great culture with no systems creates happy chaos. The vibe is good, but nothing gets done at scale. Great systems with poor culture create rigid misery. Everything looks organized, but no one wants to be there.

The sweet spot is where strong systems meet healthy culture. Where clarity and trust reinforce each other. That's when communication becomes a force for transformation. Patients feel it. Your team feels it. You feel it.

That's the practice patients never want to leave and the practice you actually want to lead.

The Communication Multiplier Effect

Consider the mathematics of effective communication: **every message properly delivered by your team without your intervention multiplies your impact.** When your front desk confidently handles insurance questions, when your assistants expertly address patient concerns about treatment options, and when your digital platforms seamlessly continue patient education after hours, you've effectively cloned your expertise without cloning yourself.

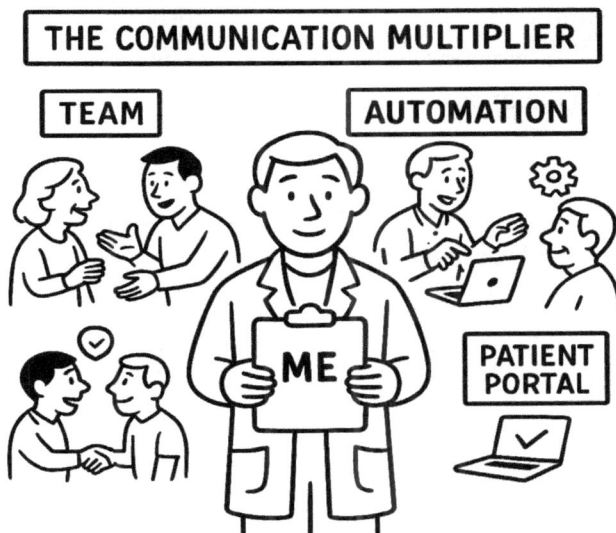

This chapter explores three critical dimensions of practice communication. First, we'll examine the fundamental communication principles that build unshakable patient trust and retention. You'll discover specific language patterns that reduce anxiety and increase case acceptance, creating the foundation for autonomous team function.

Next, we'll identify digital communication strategies that strengthen patient relationships while reducing your personal time investment. From automated follow-ups that feel genuinely personal to social media approaches that reinforce your practice values, these tools extend your communication reach without extending your workday.

Finally, we'll uncover how effective communication directly reduces practice stress while improving case acceptance rates. When information flows cleanly through your practice, resistance diminishes, efficiency increases, and your mental bandwidth expands.

The paradox resolves when we understand that relinquishing communication control, through proper systems and team empowerment, actually increases your influence and creates space for you to focus on clinical care while your team handles everything else with clarity and confidence.

The Time Freedom Paradox

Dr. Nicole sat in her office, staring at a termination notice she'd printed but hadn't signed.

Across the hall, Jess, the treatment coordinator she was ready to fire, was reviewing tomorrow's consults. Not poorly. Not exceptionally. Just... not the way Nicole would've done it. And that was the problem. Or so she thought.

The week before, Jess had mishandled a new patient intake. Missed a financial note. Fumbled through the treatment presentation. The case walked.

Nicole had been furious. She'd raised her voice. Told Jess, flat-out, "This isn't acceptable." Jess had nodded, eyes down, barely speaking. And since then, things had only gotten worse. Not because of incompetence, but because of disconnection.

Now Nicole sat with that paper in her hand and something inside her shifted.

She thought about the leadership training she'd just gone through. The lessons on rapport. On matching and mirroring. On pacing someone's emotional state before trying to lead them anywhere. She hadn't done any of that. She'd judged, reacted, and withdrawn.

She remembered how long it had taken her to learn these skills. Four years of dental school. Three years of ortho residency. Hundreds of hours in continuing education. And yet, she'd given Jess three weeks, a few checklists, and her own growing frustration.

How fair was that?

She looked out the window and took a deep breath. The real issue wasn't Jess. It was the system. The training. The communication. And most of all, the expectations that she had never taken the time to fully explain.

She stood up, walked across the hall, and sat down next to Jess.

"Can I ask you something?" she said.

Jess turned, guarded. "Of course."

"When you missed that detail last week, what was going on in your head? What were you feeling?"

Jess hesitated, then spoke. "I was overwhelmed. I didn't want to mess it up. I couldn't tell if I was supposed to just follow the script or make it more personal."

Nicole nodded. "That's on me. I didn't make it clear. And I didn't give you space to ask."

She paused. "Jess, I want this to work. But I need to start doing a better job showing you what 'right' looks like, and giving you time to get there."

It wasn't a motivational speech. It wasn't a magic moment. But it was human. And that's what had been missing.

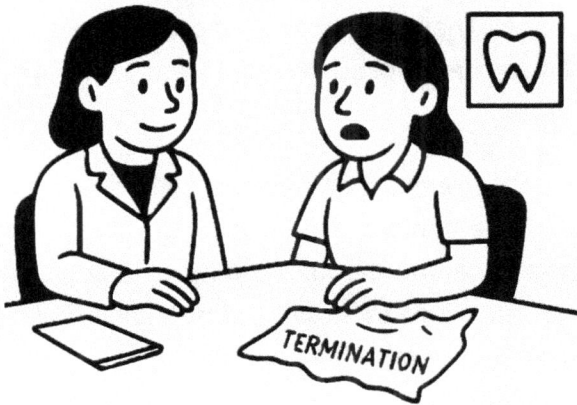

Because we forget sometimes—our team isn't behind because they don't care. They're behind because we're years ahead. And if we want them to rise, we have to meet them where they are, not where we wish they already were.

Nicole didn't lower her standards that day. She raised her communication. She led with empathy. And that's when everything started to shift.

The Foundation of Patient Trust

Communication isn't just what you say. It's what they feel when you say it.

That's the core of patient trust. It doesn't come from explanations or credentials. It comes from connection. When a patient feels understood, respected, and cared for, their defenses drop. Their trust grows. And with it, their likelihood to accept treatment, follow through, and stay loyal to your practice.

This starts with presence, or truly being with them in the room. That means eye contact. Open body language. A tone that mirrors their pace and mood. Attentive listening that doesn't just wait for your turn to speak but genuinely absorbs what they're saying—and what they're not.

Think of patient communication like tending a fire. You can light the match, but without fuel and care, it dies quickly. One rushed consult. One unanswered question. One glance at the computer while they're sharing something personal—and the warmth disappears.

TENDING THE TRUST FIRE

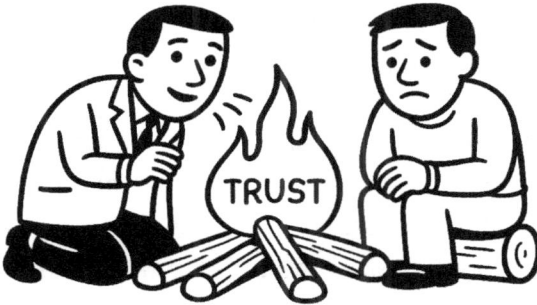

EYE CONTACT + ACTIVE LISTENING + FOLLOW-UP

And here's the reality: patients forget 80% of what you tell them. That number climbs even higher when they're nervous or overwhelmed. That's why great practices don't rely on verbal explanations alone. They reinforce with visuals, write things down, and follow up proactively. They do it because patients deserve more than just words. They deserve clarity and care at every step.

And patients notice the difference.

The best practices don't leave this to chance. They use structured communication protocols that everyone follows. From how the phone is answered to how treatment is explained to how follow-ups are managed, everything is intentional. That consistency builds more than efficiency. It builds trust.

Every interaction communicates something. Every word, every glance, every silence sends a message. The layout of your consultation room, the tone your team uses, and whether you speak while typing or turn to face the person you're serving all either reinforce confidence or quietly erode it.

And remember: people learn in different ways. Some need to see it. Some need to hear it. Some need to experience it. Great communicators adapt to the patient's rhythm in real time by mirroring their language and matching their energy. And when it's time to lead them to a decision, they do it with empathy rather than pressure.

Timing matters, too. Don't drop a $7,000 treatment plan the moment someone hears they need jaw surgery. Let it breathe. Acknowledge the emotion. Give space. That pause is not a delay. It is a gift that shows emotional intelligence and deepens trust.

And above all—connect personally. Remember names. Reference their kids. Acknowledge their fear without judgment. Be human before you're clinical. Because when patients feel that from you, they stop seeing you as a provider and start trusting you as a guide.

Masterful communication makes patients feel something real. It creates connection, builds trust, and leaves people certain they are in the right hands.

That's the foundation trust is built on. And it's worth everything.

Communication That Connects

Dental appointments come with baggage—sights, sounds, costs, and past experiences that trigger stress before a word is even spoken.

That's your reality. But it's also your opportunity.

Because communication is more than words. It is how you guide the emotional climate of the room. Every sentence, every pause, and every gesture either raises tension or brings it down. When you learn to manage that emotional thermostat, everything changes.

Stress shuts down decision-making. It clouds understanding. It breeds hesitation. If your patient is in fight-or-flight mode, chances are, they're probably not actively listening. That's why clarity, calm, and connection are non-negotiables in treatment conversations.

This isn't soft skill fluff. It's performance strategy.

Simple tone shifts. Clear, chunked information. Gentle pacing. These communication tools are often the difference between confusion and clarity, between doubt and commitment.

So if you want to increase case acceptance, start here: *lower your patients' anxiety.*

What that will require of you and your team is to ditch the rush, sit down with patients, make eye contact, and use open body language. Create the perception of time, even when the clock is tight. That perceived focus builds trust faster than any degree on the wall.

And don't just explain—frame.

Behavioral science shows us that how you present options matters as much as what the options are. Start with the comprehensive solution, then offer alternatives. When you lead with what's ideal, you define the standard.

Transparency matters, too. Don't dance around cost. Be clear and respectful, laying out the investment and the reasoning behind it. Patients are investing in outcomes, so when you connect dollars to value, you reduce fear and build belief.

And always protect autonomy. Patients don't want to be told what to do—they want to be guided toward smart choices. Use language like: "Here's what I'd recommend, and here's why. But let's talk through your goals so we find what fits you best." That one shift changes everything. It turns pressure into partnership.

Want data? Practices that train their teams in structured communication skills see 22–35% increases in case acceptance. Not through sales tactics, but through trust, rapport, and emotional intelligence.

Masterful communication reduces stress, increases clarity, builds trust, and improves decisions. That's the cycle. And it's one you control.

Not with scripts. With skill. With empathy. With presence.

The Communication Framework That Transforms Practices

If your practice grinds to a halt when you're not in the building, that's not a staffing problem. It's a systems problem, specifically a communication system problem.

Here's the goal: build a practice where your team communicates clearly, confidently, and consistently whether you're in the room or not.

Here's the framework that makes it possible:

- **Codify your core messages.** What are the 15–20 questions you get every week? Write the answers— once. Then train your team to deliver them the same way, every time. Consistency breeds clarity, and clarity builds trust.

- **Use visual tools.** Patients watch every bit as much as they listen. Equip your team with visual aids that simplify complex treatments so your message can be both seen and heard for different types of learners.

- **Build checkpoints into the patient journey.** Define when and how key communication happens—before visits, during consults, post-procedure. Don't leave this to chance. Automate the rhythm, then humanize the delivery.

- **Train active listeners.** Teach your team to listen for what's said—and what isn't. Nonverbals, hesitation, tone. The best communicators hear beneath the words.

- **Establish real feedback loops.** Ask for input. Make it easy. And more importantly—do something with it. When patients feel heard, they stay. When team members feel heard, they grow.

- **Empower through decision trees.** Don't just tell your team *what not to do*. Show them what they *can do* without asking. Confidence rises when the path is clear.

- **Rehearse hard conversations.** Don't wait for the real moment to practice. Role-play the tough stuff—money talk, delays, dissatisfaction. Confidence is built in the reps.

Following these tips the right way will make your team communications systems scalable without micromanaging their every move.

When one client of ours implemented this framework, her treatment coordinators went from handling 40% of new consults independently to over 90%. As patient satisfaction shot through the roof, stress levels fell in an equal and opposite response, putting several hours per week back into her schedule. She used that time to focus on complex cases and real leadership.

That's the shift: communication moves from being a bottleneck to becoming a system that works for you.

When it's built right:

- Your team leads with confidence, not hesitation.

- Patients feel heard and informed at every step.

- You're no longer the glue holding everything together.

The Communication Mastery Blueprint

Goal: Shift from clinician-dependent to team-empowered communication, allowing your practice to operate on clarity rather than constant oversight.

1. Audit the Now (1–2 Days)

Pull real examples from recent patient interactions, highlighting where things worked and where they didn't. Don't sugarcoat: growth starts with truth, and you can't fix blind spots you're afraid to look at.

2. Implement Active Listening (1 Week)

This week, slow down. Hold eye contact. Nod with intent. Resist the urge to interrupt or "fix" too quickly. Jot down what changed. You'll be surprised what people tell you when they feel safe enough to speak.

3. Build a Question Bank (2–3 Days)

Open-ended questions unlock understanding. Create a list your whole team can use: "What concerns you most about this treatment?" "How are you feeling about today's visit?" Practice them until they feel natural, then embed them into your culture.

4. Use Tech That Feels Human (2 Weeks)

Choose digital tools that reinforce—not replace—relationships. Prioritize systems that automate logistics (reminders, follow-ups) while preserving your tone and care. Train your team, test it yourself, then go live.

5. Personalize On Purpose (Ongoing)

Track the details: hobbies, family, life updates. Reference them in real conversations. Patients want to feel seen as well as heard, and building these real connections are the first step toward doing just that.

6. Ask for Feedback (Monthly)

Create a 2–3 question feedback form post-visit: "Did you feel heard?" "Was anything unclear?" Review monthly as a team. Use what you learn. Close the loop.

7. Measure Autonomy Gains (Quarterly)

Track what matters: fewer clinical interruptions, more team-led consults, fewer after-hours calls. These metrics provide proof your leadership is scaling.

Here's the paradox: the better your communication, the less you're needed. Not because you've checked out—but because your team has leveled up.

That's the shift.

When your patients trust your team as much as they trust you...

When your systems communicate while you sleep...

When clarity prevents chaos...

That's when you stop being the bottleneck—and start being the builder.

Mastery is not about perfection. It is about building progress that continues even when you are not holding everything together.

Start with the areas where you struggle most. Apply this blueprint consistently and see what happens as trust grows and burnout fades.

You do not have to carry the weight alone. When communication is done right, it carries part of the load for you.

One day, you will leave on time with your phone quiet, inbox calm, and practice thriving, and you will know this was the lever that made it possible.

Key Takeaways

- Communication is not just words. It's how trust, culture, and freedom are built.

- Great systems without culture create rigidity; great culture without systems creates chaos. Transformation happens when both align.

- Patients don't remember most of what you say, but they always remember how you made them feel. Communication must reinforce clarity and care at every step.

- Scaling your practice requires systems that allow your team to communicate effectively without you in the room.

- Masterful communication reduces stress, increases case acceptance, and gives you back time and freedom.

Next Steps

You don't have to build a perfect system overnight. Starting this week, you can:

Listen with intention – Slow down in one key patient or team interaction. Focus on hearing not just the words, but the emotions and concerns behind them.

Codify one message – Choose a recurring question or issue in your practice (billing, scheduling, treatment explanation) and write down a clear, consistent answer your team can use.

Notice your defaults – Pay attention to moments when you jump in to "fix" communication. Ask yourself: *Is this about clarity, or about control?* Use it as a chance to lead with trust.

Communication is the lifeblood of your practice. Clarity and systems are integral to delegating and making yourself replaceable. The next step is building **meaningful relationships**. Communication is the tool, but relationships are the outcome. In Chapter 3, we'll explore how to move beyond transactions and build the kind of connections that make your team unstoppable and your patients fiercely loyal.

Chapter 3: Building Meaningful Relationships

By: Luke Infinger

The Weight of Minutes

Dr. Eleanor glanced at her watch—already ten minutes behind, and only her third patient of the morning. The clinic schedule gave her fifteen minutes with Mrs. Garner, but Eleanor knew the visit would take twice that long. Mrs. Garner's list of health issues was complex, and her anxious eyes always pleaded for more than a rushed answer. Eleanor wanted to slow down, to truly listen—but the weight of the clock pressed against her chest.

The system told her to move faster. Her heart told her to pause. And in that tension, she felt the quiet ache of a truth too many clinicians ignore: if patients don't feel heard, communication fails before it even begins.

At the heart of every sustainable, fulfilling practice are strong relationships. When you feel forced to choose between speed and connection, you lose both. However, when you intentionally invest in meaningful relationships with patients, colleagues, and mentors, you not only improve clinical outcomes and foster practice growth, but you also rediscover the deeper purpose that drew you to healthcare in the first place.

This chapter is about transforming communication into connection and connection into care that lasts. You'll see how building meaningful relationships doesn't just strengthen patient trust; it creates resilient teams, fosters supportive mentorship, and anchors you in a professional community that keeps burnout at bay.

The Relationship Crisis Hiding in Plain Sight

Time is the currency of human connection. In today's healthcare environment, clinicians frequently find themselves trapped in a cycle that demands impossible choices: see more patients or provide better care. This false dichotomy lies at the heart of what I call the practice paradox. The truth is that meaningful relationships with colleagues, mentors, and patients are essential foundations for both professional excellence and personal wellbeing.

The mathematics of modern practice can frequently feel unforgiving. When you're scheduled to see patients every fifteen minutes, something has to give. Too often, it's the quality of interaction that suffers. A clinician rushing from room to room barely maintains eye contact, misses subtle cues, and leaves both parties feeling shortchanged. The irony? This rushed approach ultimately creates more work through misdiagnoses, patient dissatisfaction, and the emotional toll of performing below your own standards.

Relationship-centered care isn't just better for patients—it's better for you. The evidence is clear: clinicians who build meaningful connections with patients experience greater job satisfaction and lower burnout rates. When you take time to listen, explain, and connect, you not only deliver better clinical outcomes but also nurture the very reason most of us entered healthcare in the first place, to make a difference in people's lives.

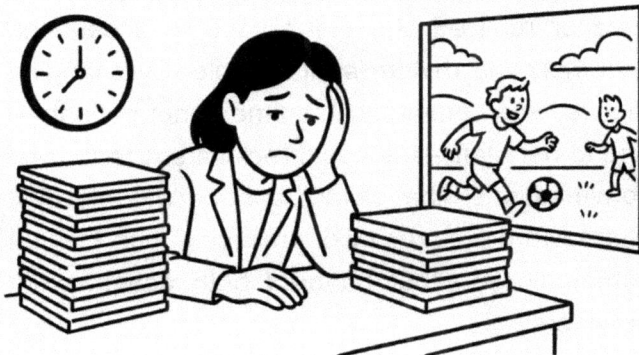

THE WEIGHT OF MINUTES

The Weight of Minutes Continued Later that afternoon, Eleanor stared at Mrs. Garner's chart still open on her desk. The visit had run long, the schedule was wrecked, and she knew she'd be staying late again. But what weighed on her wasn't the paperwork piling up—it was the memory of Mrs. Garner's eyes, searching for reassurance that couldn't fit into a fifteen-minute slot. The thought of her own grandmother came rushing back—how rushed appointments and missed signs had cost her life. Eleanor felt the same trap tightening around her now: a system designed for speed, not care. She reached for the phone. "Janet," she said to the clinic manager, her voice steady, "I need to talk about restructuring my schedule. Today, not next week." In that moment, something shifted. Eleanor realized she didn't have to accept the assembly-line rhythm as inevitable. By changing the way she communicated time to her patients— and to her staff—she could reclaim space for real conversations. That call to Janet became her first step toward a new way of practicing: one built on communication that honored both patients and providers.

The Three Critical Relationships in Professional Practice

Every successful dental or orthodontic practice is built on three essential relationships: with patients, peers, and mentors. These connections shape not only how you deliver care, but how you sustain your own well-being, growth, and purpose.

Your **relationship with patients** is the foundation. Every interaction builds or erodes trust. When patients feel truly seen and heard, they engage more deeply in their care. Compliance improves, outcomes strengthen, and satisfaction grows. More importantly, you reconnect with the human side of healthcare: trust, empathy, and respect.

Your **relationship with your professional network** keeps you connected and supported. Isolation is one of the quietest threats to clinician satisfaction. By staying engaged with colleagues and peers, you gain perspective, share wisdom, and find resilience in a demanding profession.

Your **relationship with mentors** accelerates growth. A great mentor offers perspective that experience alone cannot provide, challenging assumptions, offering guidance, and expanding your vision. Mentorship is also reciprocal: when you mentor others, you strengthen your own mastery and contribute to the profession's growth.

Together, these three relationships form an ecosystem that sustains your purpose and success. In the sections that follow, we will explore each one, how to build it, how to sustain it, and how to make it the cornerstone of a fulfilling, balanced practice.

1. Patient Relationships

The Patient Connection

Patient relationships form the foundation of healthcare practice. Clinical expertise alone doesn't guarantee practice success—the quality of your patient connections determines both satisfaction and outcomes. Research consistently demonstrates that patients who feel genuinely seen and heard comply better with treatment plans and report higher satisfaction regardless of clinical outcomes.

Creating these connections requires more than technical competence. It demands presence. When patients enter your office, they bring not just symptoms but fears, expectations, and personal stories. The clinician who addresses only the clinical presentation misses crucial context that could inform better care. Taking time to listen—truly listen—differentiates a transaction from a healing relationship.

Think of patient interactions as conversations rather than consultations. In a good conversation, both parties contribute and feel valued. Similarly, the most effective patient relationships involve collaboration rather than dictation. When patients participate actively in their care

PRESENCE OVER PERFORMANCE

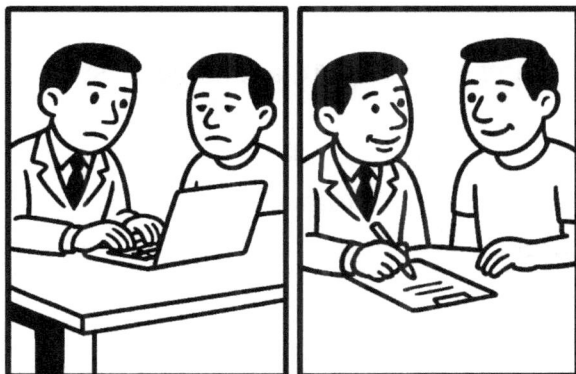

decisions, they develop greater ownership of their health journey and stronger trust in your guidance.

Technology has introduced new challenges to authentic patient connection. Electronic health records and practice management systems increase efficiency but can create barriers between clinicians and patients. The clinician focused on a computer screen rather than making eye contact signals divided attention. Balancing technological tools with human connection requires conscious effort but yields substantial benefits.

Non-verbal communication speaks volumes in patient interactions. Your body language, facial expressions, and tone convey more about your attentiveness than your words. Patients instinctively sense whether you're fully present or mentally rushing to the next appointment. Simple adjustments such as sitting rather than standing, maintaining eye contact, and nodding in acknowledgment signal genuine engagement and build trust.

The time constraints of modern practice create pressure to abbreviate patient interactions. This efficiency-driven approach often backfires, as rushed appointments lead to missed information, repeated visits, and diminished satisfaction. Restructuring schedules to allow adequate time for each patient may seem counterintuitive from a business perspective but often improves both clinical outcomes and practice profitability through better retention and referrals.

Cultural competence enhances patient connection. As communities grow more diverse, clinicians must develop awareness of how cultural backgrounds influence health beliefs, communication styles, and treatment preferences. This understanding isn't about stereotyping but rather approaching each patient with respectful curiosity about their unique perspective. The clinician who acknowledges cultural differences while avoiding assumptions creates space for authentic connection.

Building meaningful patient relationships requires balancing professional expertise with personal warmth, technological efficiency with human connection, and clinical protocols with individual needs. These relationships not only improve patient outcomes but also create the professional fulfillment that sustains clinicians throughout their careers. When we connect authentically with patients, we create the foundation for both clinical success and leadership development, while mentorship relationships accelerate our growth in these critical interpersonal skills.

The Art of Patient Connection

Authentic patient relationships begin with presence. Before addressing clinical concerns, take a moment to truly see the person before you. Simple acknowledgments—using preferred names, referencing previous conversations, noting important life events—signal that you recognize the individual beyond their medical chart. These small gestures create the foundation for meaningful connection.

Time pressures present the greatest barrier to patient connection. When clinicians feel rushed, patients sense the hurry and hesitate to share important information. Restructuring appointment scheduling to allow adequate time—even if it means seeing fewer patients daily—often improves both care quality and clinician satisfaction. This adjustment may initially seem financially counterintuitive but typically pays dividends through improved retention and word-of-mouth referrals.

Connection happens through conversation, not interrogation. Clinical questionnaires gather necessary data but rarely build relationships. Balancing structured assessment with open-ended questions allows patients to share what matters most to them. Simple prompts like "What concerns you most about this situation?" or "How is this affecting your daily life?" invite meaningful dialogue beyond symptom reports.

Patient education becomes more effective within established relationships. When patients trust your concern for their well-being, they become more receptive to recommendations and more likely to implement suggested changes. The time invested in connection often returns multiplied benefits through improved compliance and outcomes.

Strengthening the Patient Connection

Patient relationships begin before the first meeting. Review information beforehand to demonstrate preparation and respect for their time. This simple practice shifts the initial interaction from information gathering to connection building. Patients notice the difference between clinicians who start from scratch and those who arrive already familiar with their situation.

Consider Your Office Environment

The appointment environment has a significant impact on connection quality. Consider factors beyond basic comfort, such as privacy that allows for vulnerable sharing, seating arrangements that facilitate conversation rather than examination, and minimal distractions that enable full attention. These environmental elements communicate your priorities more clearly than verbal assurances.

Make a Good First Impression

First impressions establish relationship trajectories. Simple courtesies, such as punctuality, introducing all team members, and explaining what to expect, create a foundation of respect. Address patients by their preferred names and pronouns—these basic acknowledgments of individuality signal recognition of the person beyond their clinical presentation.

Speak with Clarity & Empathy

Language choices shape patient experiences. Technical terminology creates distance while accessible explanations build understanding. Notice when patients appear confused and adjust accordingly. Remember that stress and anxiety impair information processing—concepts clear to you may need multiple explanations in different formats for patient comprehension.

Be an Active Listener

Listen for what remains unsaid. Patients often hint at concerns rather than stating them directly, particularly when discussing sensitive topics or fearing judgment. Skilled clinicians develop an awareness of these subtle signals and create opportunities for fuller expression. Simple prompts, such as "Is there anything else on your mind?" can invite essential revelations.

Develop Cultural Awareness

Cultural humility enhances connection across differences. Rather than assuming understanding of cultural factors, approach each patient with genuine curiosity about their unique perspective and preferences. This stance acknowledges the limitations of general cultural knowledge while demonstrating respect for individual experience. The question "How does your family/ community typically approach this kind of situation?" often reveals important context.

Create Space for Shared Decision-Making

Shared decision-making transforms the clinician-patient dynamic. When patients actively participate in treatment planning, they develop greater ownership of their health outcomes and stronger trust in the therapeutic relationship. This approach requires more time initially but typically improves compliance and satisfaction. The clinician becomes a trusted advisor rather than an authoritarian director.

Keep Your Commitments

Follow-through strengthens trust. When you promise to research a question, check on a referral, or provide additional information, reliable delivery on these commitments builds credibility. Conversely, even minor lapses in follow-through can undermine the quality of a relationship. Establish systems that ensure you fulfill every promise made to patients.

The same principles that strengthen patient relationships—presence, empathy, and communication—also
apply to how you connect with your peers. While patient care provides meaning, professional connection offers strength. Many clinicians find that as their practice
grows, so does a quiet sense of isolation. The next step
in building a sustainable, fulfilling career lies in cultivating professional networks that offer support, perspective,
and shared wisdom. These relationships form the back-
bone of collaboration and growth, ensuring that you don't
have to navigate the complexities of practice alone.

---

2. Professional Networks

The Leadership Paradox

Healthcare leadership brings immense responsibility.
When you're at the helm of a practice, decisions rest
on your shoulders. Patient care, staff management, and
business operations all demand your attention daily. This
position of authority often creates an unexpected side
effect: isolation. Many clinicians find themselves feeling
alone despite being surrounded by people all day.

Think of leadership as standing on a mountaintop. The view is expansive and you can see far in all directions, but the air is thin and few others share your space. Those who haven't climbed the same peak may not understand the challenges you face or the decisions you must make. This isolation is emotionally taxing, and even worse, it can impair your effectiveness as both a leader and a clinician.

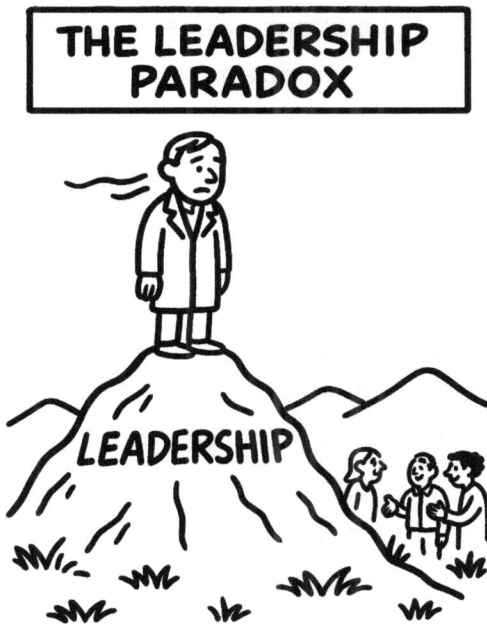

THE LEADERSHIP PARADOX

LEADERSHIP

Professional networks serve as the antidote to leadership isolation. They connect you with peers facing similar challenges and opportunities. Research consistently shows that healthcare clinicians with strong professional connections report higher job satisfaction and lower burnout rates. These networks provide sounding boards for ideas, validation for concerns, and fresh perspectives on persistent problems.

Building these connections requires intentional effort. Professional associations, conferences, and continuing education events provide natural venues for meeting colleagues. Digital platforms have expanded networking possibilities, allowing clinicians to connect regardless of geographic limitations. The investment in these relationships pays dividends through enhanced problem-solving capabilities and emotional support during difficult times.

Many healthcare leaders mistakenly believe that strength means solving problems independently. This mindset creates unnecessary stress and limits access to collective wisdom. The most effective leaders recognize that vulnerability and connection lead to better outcomes. Sharing challenges with trusted colleagues often reveals solutions you might never have considered on your own.

Professional networks also expand your practice's capabilities. No single clinician can specialize in everything. Developing relationships with complementary specialists creates referral pathways that benefit your patients while strengthening your professional community. These mutually beneficial relationships improve care quality while distributing the burden of comprehensive treatment.

The paradox of healthcare leadership is that strength comes not from isolation but from meaningful connection with others who understand your unique challenges.

Networks That Nurture Growth

Professional isolation doesn't happen overnight. It develops gradually as clinicians focus intensely on their immediate responsibilities. Days filled with patient care, staff management, and administrative tasks leave little energy for external connections. Before long, what began as dedication becomes unintentional isolation.

The consequences extend beyond emotional well-being. Isolated clinicians lack exposure to evolving best practices and innovative approaches. They miss opportunities for collaboration that could enhance patient care and practice efficiency. Without an external perspective, they may continue outdated methods simply because alternatives remain unknown.

"In healthcare, the lone wolf rarely thrives for long," notes Dr. Paul Grundy, founding president of the Patient-Centered Primary Care Collaborative. "The complexity of modern medicine demands collective wisdom and mutual support." This observation highlights how professional networks serve both practical and emotional needs at once.

Building these connections doesn't require overwhelming time commitments. Even brief, consistent engagement with professional communities yields benefits. Monthly association meetings, quarterly study groups, or annual conferences can maintain vital connections. The key lies in prioritizing these interactions rather than treating them as optional extras when time permits.

Within every strong professional network lies the potential for something more profound: mentorship. While networks provide breadth in connection, collaboration, and shared experience, mentorship offers depth. It transforms casual professional relationships into purposeful partnerships focused on growth. The following section explores how mentors help you navigate challenges, accelerate development, and expand what's possible in both your practice and your career.

3. Mentor Relationships

The Mentorship Advantage

Mentorship accelerates growth in ways that solo learning simply cannot. Those who benefit from strong mentor relationships gain access to hard-won wisdom, avoiding common pitfalls and discovering efficient paths forward. The right mentor offers more than technical advice. They help you navigate the unwritten rules of practice management, challenge your assumptions, and expand your vision of what is possible.

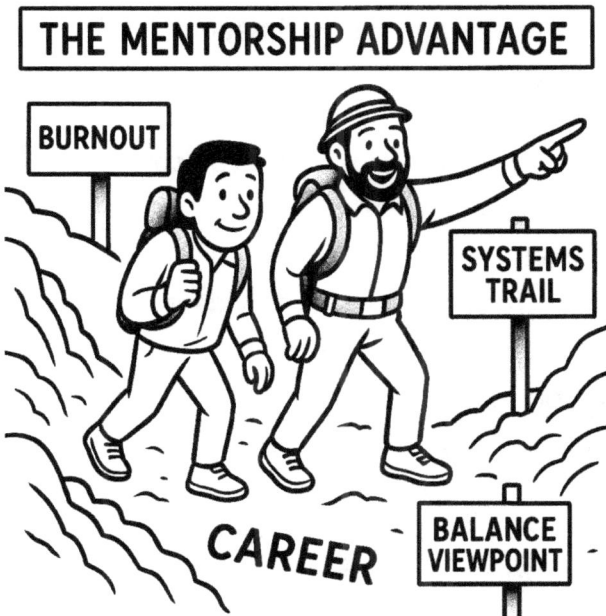

THE MENTORSHIP ADVANTAGE

BURNOUT

SYSTEMS TRAIL

CAREER

BALANCE VIEWPOINT

Mentorship accelerates professional growth in ways that independent learning cannot match. The guidance of someone who has navigated similar challenges offers valuable insights and shortcuts through the complexity of healthcare practice management. In fact, research shows that clinicians with mentors reach proficiency faster and report greater confidence in their clinical and business decisions.

What makes mentorship different from other professional relationships? The depth and intentionality. While networking creates broad connections, mentorship develops deep relationships focused on your specific growth. Mentors invest personally in your development, offering tailored advice and feedback based on your unique situation and goals.

Finding the right mentor is akin to discovering a guide for an unfamiliar wilderness. You wouldn't choose someone who's never traversed the terrain. Similarly, effective mentors have successfully navigated the challenges you're facing. Their experience becomes your roadmap, helping you avoid common pitfalls while highlighting opportunities you might otherwise miss.

The mentorship relationship requires vulnerability and a willingness to be humble. Exposing your uncertainties and areas for growth can feel uncomfortable, especially for healthcare clinicians accustomed to projecting confidence. Yet this openness creates the conditions for meaningful guidance. The most valuable mentoring moments often emerge from honest discussions about struggles rather than celebrations of success.

Truly effective mentorship also involves both structured interactions and spontaneous guidance. Regular meetings provide opportunities to discuss specific challenges and progress toward goals. Meanwhile, real-time advice during unexpected situations often delivers the most impactful learning opportunities. The balance between these formal and informal exchanges creates a comprehensive development experience.

Many clinicians mistakenly believe they should have outgrown the need for mentorship by mid-career. This misconception limits continued growth. The most successful healthcare leaders maintain mentorship relationships throughout their careers, adapting the focus as their needs evolve. Early-career mentorship may emphasize clinical skills and practice management, while established clinicians benefit from mentors who guide them in advanced business strategy or work-life integration.

Mentorship also creates a legacy of knowledge transfer within the healthcare profession. When you benefit from mentorship, you develop the capacity to mentor others.

This cycle ensures that valuable experiential knowledge is passed from generation to generation, thereby strengthening the profession as a whole. Many clinicians find that serving as mentors becomes one of the most rewarding aspects of their careers.

The digital age has expanded mentorship possibilities beyond geographic limitations. Virtual mentorship enables clinicians to connect with ideal guides, regardless of their location. These relationships may lack the spontaneity of in-person interactions, but they compensate by allowing connections that would otherwise be impossible to form. The key lies in maintaining regular and meaningful communication, despite the distance.

What might change in your practice if you approached each challenge with not only your wisdom but also the accumulated insights of someone who has successfully navigated similar terrain?

The Mentor's Roadmap

Mentorship transforms abstract knowledge into practical wisdom. While education provides the foundation of healthcare practice, mentorship teaches the nuanced application of that knowledge in real-world situations. This guidance becomes particularly valuable when navigating complex decisions without clear textbook answers.

The mentor-mentee relationship thrives on clear expectations. Effective mentorship begins with honest conversation about goals, communication preferences, and time commitments. Without this foundation, mismatched expectations can undermine otherwise valuable connections. Take time to establish mutual understanding before diving into specific challenges.

"Show me a successful person in any field, and I'll show you someone who had real positive influences in their life," says basketball coach Phil Jackson. While speaking about sports, his observation applies equally to healthcare. Success rarely develops in isolation; it grows through guidance, challenge, and support from those who recognize potential and nurture growth.

Effective mentees demonstrate specific qualities. They approach the relationship with curiosity rather than defensiveness, seeking understanding rather than validation. They follow through on suggestions and report outcomes, creating a feedback loop that refines future guidance. They respect their mentor's time while making the most of available learning opportunities.

The mentorship journey evolves. Early interactions may focus on specific technical challenges or immediate decisions. As trust builds, conversations often shift toward broader questions of professional identity, leadership philosophy, and long-term vision. This evolution keeps the relationship relevant throughout career transitions and prevents stagnation.

Many clinicians benefit from having multiple mentors address different aspects of their professional development. A clinical mentor might guide treatment approaches while a business mentor advises on practice management. A work-life integration mentor could help navigate the personal challenges of a demanding profession. This constellation of guidance offers comprehensive support that surpasses what any single mentor could provide.

Mentorship extends beyond formal arrangements. Observational learning—watching how experienced clinicians handle difficult situations—provides valuable education even without explicit teaching. Pay attention to how respected colleagues communicate with patients, manage staff conflicts, or approach complex cases. These observations complement direct guidance.

The most valuable mentorship often emerges during challenging situations. When facing difficult decisions or recovering from mistakes, the mentor's perspective provides both practical guidance and emotional support. These moments—though uncomfortable—frequently generate the most significant professional growth and the deepest mentoring connections.

Mentor Relationships in Practice

Identifying potential mentors requires both self-awareness and environmental scanning. Begin by clarifying your development needs and professional aspirations. Then observe who demonstrates mastery in these areas. Effective mentors typically share some similarities with you—enough for mutual understanding—while bringing different perspectives or experiences that enrich your thinking.

Approaching potential mentors deserves thoughtful preparation. Rather than requesting a vague mentoring relationship, start with specific, limited interactions. Request guidance on a specific challenge or receive feedback on a particular project. These focused exchanges allow both parties to assess compatibility before committing to ongoing involvement.

Consider creating a personal board of advisors rather than seeking a single all-purpose mentor. This approach acknowledges that different individuals bring unique strengths to the development process. One person might excel at clinical reasoning, another at business strategy, and another at navigating institutional politics. Together, they provide comprehensive guidance that no individual could offer alone.

Reciprocity strengthens mentoring relationships. While mentees naturally receive more guidance than they give, look for opportunities to contribute value. This might involve research assistance, technology support, or simply demonstrated implementation of advice received. These contributions honor the mentor's investment and create more balanced interaction.

Formal mentorship programs offer structured entry points for these relationships. Many professional associations, healthcare institutions, and educational organizations maintain such programs. These structured approaches provide clear parameters and expectations, reducing the awkwardness sometimes associated with initiating mentoring connections independently.

Virtual mentorship expands possibilities beyond geographic limitations. When local options don't match your specific needs, consider remote relationships facilitated through video calls and digital communication. These connections lack some of the benefits of in-person interaction, but they enable access to expertise that would otherwise be unavailable. The key lies in establishing regular, meaningful communication despite the distance.

Document your learning from mentorship interactions. Brief reflections on insights gained and actions taken help integrate guidance into practice. These notes also serve as valuable reference material for future situations. The documentation process itself deepens learning by requiring articulation of sometimes tacit understanding.

Cultivating Your Professional Ecosystem

Patient relationships, professional networks, and mentorships require intentional cultivation and nurturing. Consider scheduling regular time for professional connection just as you would for continuing education or administrative tasks. This deliberate approach prevents relationship-building from becoming an afterthought addressed only when immediate needs arise.

The investment yields compound returns. Strong professional relationships create resilience during challenging periods. When facing difficult decisions, practice transitions, or personal struggles, these connections provide both emotional support and practical assistance. They transform potential crisis points into growth opportunities through shared wisdom and encouragement.

Technology offers both opportunities and challenges for relationship development. Digital platforms expand connection possibilities but can create false impressions of depth. Remember that liking posts or exchanging brief messages differs fundamentally from conversations that build genuine understanding. Use technology as a supplement to, not a replacement for, meaningful interaction.

Balance your relationship portfolio just as financial advisors recommend diversified investments, professional development benefits from varied connections. Seek relationships with both peers and those at different career stages. Include people within your specialty and those with complementary expertise. This diversity provides a broader perspective than any homogeneous group could offer.

The quality of your professional relationships significantly influences career satisfaction. Research consistently shows that clinicians with strong connection networks report greater fulfillment and resilience regardless of other workplace factors. These relationships provide the context in which technical excellence becomes meaningful service rather than isolated performance.

The relationships you build determine both your impact and your satisfaction as a healthcare clinician. **Professional networks prevent the isolation that leads to stagnation and burnout. Mentorship relationships accelerate your growth through others' wisdom. Patient connections transform technical service into meaningful care.** Together, these relationships create the context in which both clinical excellence and personal fulfillment flourish.

The Relationship Advantage

Building meaningful relationships is crucial to establishing a sustainable practice that benefits both you and your patients. Throughout this chapter, we've explored how authentic connections transform the daily experience of practicing medicine.

When you step back from the constant rush of appointments and paperwork, you'll notice that the quality of your professional life directly correlates with the quality of your relationships. Those who thrive in healthcare have mastered this fundamental truth.

Your patient relationships ultimately determine the success of your practice. By creating systems that facilitate genuine connections during appointments, you transform routine clinical encounters into meaningful exchanges. Patients who feel truly seen and heard become partners in their care rather than passive recipients.

The mentors who guide your journey offer more than just technical knowledge. They provide wisdom that can save you years of trial and error. Rather than viewing mentorship as simply receiving advice, approach it as an active, evolving partnership that demands your engagement and commitment.

Remember that professional isolation doesn't have to be your reality. The networks you cultivate not only provide clinical insights but also create the support system necessary for navigating the complexities of healthcare leadership. These connections become your sounding board, your reality check, and often, your path to innovation.

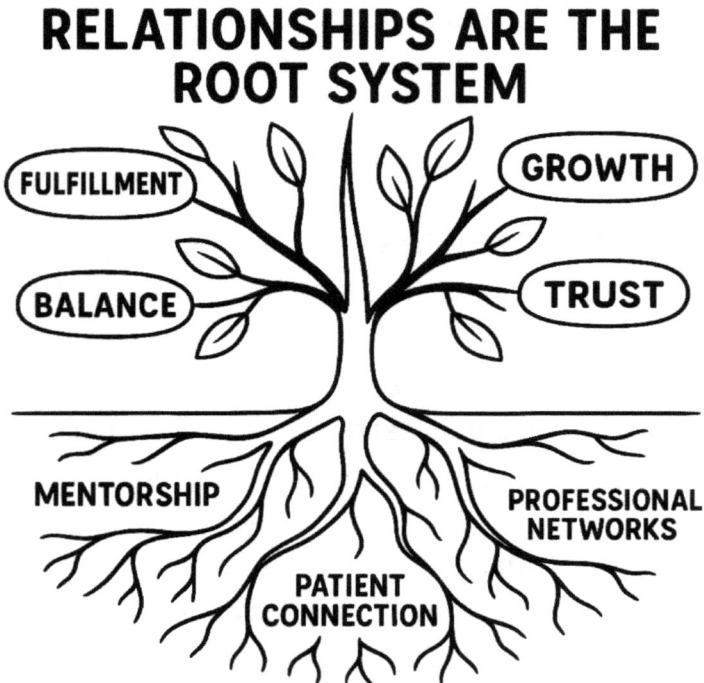

RELATIONSHIPS ARE THE ROOT SYSTEM

FULFILLMENT

GROWTH

BALANCE

TRUST

MENTORSHIP

PROFESSIONAL NETWORKS

PATIENT CONNECTION

Prioritize relationships as a cornerstone of practice management, not as an afterthought. Create systems that protect time for meaningful connection. Recognize that the moments spent deepening professional relationships and genuinely connecting with patients aren't distractions from your work; they are your work, in its most essential form.

Keep in mind that balancing excellent patient care with personal sustainability isn't just possible, it's necessary. The relationships you nurture become the infrastructure that supports everything else you hope to accomplish in your practice and your life.

Key Takeaways

- Time pressures create a false choice between efficiency and connection; meaningful relationships actually improve both.

- Professional isolation is dangerous—networks and mentors provide resilience, perspective, and growth.

- Patient relationships thrive on presence, empathy, and cultural awareness, not just technical expertise.

- Mentorship and networking accelerate growth and prevent burnout by sharing wisdom and support.

Next Steps

Start building better relationships this week:

Prioritize presence in one interaction – Slow down and give full attention to one patient, team member, or peer without watching the clock.

Reach out to a colleague or mentor – Reconnect with someone in your professional network for perspective and support.

Choose one relationship to intentionally strengthen – Whether with a patient, team member, or peer- and focus on small, consistent actions that build trust over the next 30 days.

The relationships you want to build can only thrive if the practice itself fits who you are. Communication and trust matter, but if your practice model is misaligned with your personality and lifestyle, even the best relationships will suffer.

The next step is understanding your practice personality type. The model you choose shapes the patients you attract, the culture your team experiences, and the way you spend your days. In the next chapter, we'll uncover the six practice personality types and help you decide if the practice you're running is truly the one that fits you.

Section III: Identity & Leadership

Discover:

Chapter 4 – Practice Personality Types: How aligning your practice model with your authentic self creates both freedom and sustainability.

Chapter 5 – Team Culture and Leadership: How empowering your team with trust and leadership transforms your culture into the foundation of freedom.

Chapter 4:
Practice Personality Types

By: Dr. Kyle Fagala

When Dr. Emily bought her practice, she thought she was stepping into stability. The systems were already in place, the schedule was full, and on paper, everything looked like success. But almost immediately, she realized something was wrong. The previous doctor's model ran on grueling hours—first exam at 7 AM, last at 5 PM, with patients squeezed in on alternating Fridays. For Emily, who had just learned she was pregnant with her first child, the schedule didn't just feel exhausting; It felt impossible. She wasn't just inheriting a practice; she was inheriting someone else's life.

Your practice has a personality, whether you've chosen it or not. When that personality aligns with your values, strengths, and lifestyle, everything falls into place—your team culture, patient relationships, and even your marketing. When it doesn't, no amount of hard work or money will fix the friction. Alignment between who you are and how you practice is the foundation of sustainable success.

Relationships can't thrive if the practice itself is misaligned with who you are. Your team and patients experience your practice model every day. If it doesn't fit you, it won't fit them either.

Your practice personality type is not just a business model; it's your professional DNA. And when it matches your authentic self, your practice stops being a prison and becomes an expression of your purpose.

This chapter examines six practice personality types that we have consistently noticed among doctor owners. You'll learn how to identify your type, how to adapt when your life season changes, and how misalignment can lead to burnout. Most importantly, you'll see how intentionally choosing a practice personality creates a foundation for fulfillment for you, your team, and your patients.

Your Practice Has a Personality Problem

Here's the brutal truth: Most dentists and orthodontists are running practices that don't fit who they are.

They've inherited someone else's model. Copied a mentor's approach. Or worse—they're trying to be everything to everyone, which means they're nothing to anyone. The result is burnout, misaligned patients, marketing that doesn't work, and a practice that feels like a prison instead of an expression of purpose.

But here's what the successful ones have figured out:

Your practice personality type isn't just a business model—it's your professional DNA.

When you align who you are with how you practice, everything changes. Your marketing becomes authentic. Your patients become advocates. Your team gets it. And you stop fighting yourself every single day.

The Work-Life Integration Revolution

Forget work-life balance. That's old thinking.

The rigid divide between professional and personal life is dead. It was killing dentists anyway—this constant compartmentalization that turns life into a series of competing priorities.

The new model supports **integration, not segregation.**

The most fulfilled clinicians don't separate their existence into neat "work" and "life" containers. They've designed practices that complement their personal priorities rather than compete with them. That means developing a practice that fits your life requires you to intentionally craft a practice personality type that honors who you are as a complete human being.

When your practice serves your life instead of stealing from it, everything shifts.

The Moment of Truth

Dr. Emily began to notice the ripple effects immediately. Her staff, many of whom drove more than 30 minutes to work, were exhausted. Turnover was a persistent issue, and morale suffered as a result. Even with a nanny, Emily knew what her team was facing: the stress of waking young children at 6 AM, struggling to find early daycare, and juggling family commitments that the practice hours simply didn't respect.

She realized she had a choice. She could continue down the path she inherited, grinding herself and her staff into resentment—or she could rebuild the practice around the life and relationships she wanted to sustain.

So she made a bold decision. Emily shifted her hours to 8:30–4:00, twelve clinical days per month. No more dawn appointments. No more late evenings. No more inherited compromises. At first, she feared patients might leave and production would fall. Instead, the opposite happened. Her staff became happier, her team more stable, and over the next decade, her practice grew almost fourfold.

> Her insight was simple but profound: success isn't about mimicking someone else's model—it's about creating one that reflects who you are and the life you want to live.

The Six Practice Personality Types That Actually Work

We've analyzed thousands of practices. Worked with clinicians across all 50 states. And here's what we've discovered:

There are six distinct practice personality types that consistently create both professional success and personal fulfillment.

Most clinicians get trapped in identities they've inherited rather than chosen. They operate within structures created by mentors, partners, or industry expectations—instead of intentionally designing a practice that reflects their unique combination of talents, values, and life circumstances.

This misalignment is what creates burnout.

Your practice personality type determines everything: how you serve patients, how you market, how you hire, how you spend your days. When these elements align with who you actually are, friction disappears and effectiveness multiplies.

The magic happens when your practice identity evolves with your life seasons. A model that works brilliantly in your early career might become unbearable when children arrive or as your priorities shift.

The most overlooked skill in dentistry? The ability to intentionally evolve your practice personality type.

Marketing Reality Check

Here's something most consultants and industry experts won't tell you:

Your practice personality type determines which marketing actually works.

Each personality type attracts different patients who value different things.

For example, High-Volume Clinics and Multi-Location Empires thrive on Facebook ads because their ideal patients make decisions through community recommendations. But Tech-Forward and Boutique practices often pour money into Facebook with disappointing results. Their patients aren't scrolling social media for healthcare decisions—they're researching "3D orthodontic imaging" on Google at 11 PM.

It seems self-evident, but you must match your marketing spend to how your ideal patients actually make decisions.

We'll briefly cover this for each practice personality type below, providing 3-tier recommendations for Meta Ads, Google Ads, and web presence (including initial website and ongoing SEO investments).

1. The Tech-Forward Office

Marketing Focus: Low Meta, Medium Google, Medium Web

The bleeding edge of dental innovation. These practices attract patients who value the latest technology, advanced treatment options, and modern approaches to care.

Dr. Jason Yang exemplifies this persona with his practice in the suburbs of Philadelphia. When he took over, it still operated with paper charts and traditional impressions—structured more around orthodontist efficiency than a patient-centered experience. From the beginning, he set out to reimagine the entire model into something more personalized, premium, and modern.

"Over time, I invested heavily in technology—integrating CBCT imaging, 3D printing, and clinical systems that allow us to routinely perform advanced procedures like MARPEs, TADs, and gingivectomies," Dr. Yang explains. "Initially, these upgrades came with the pressure to increase volume just to justify the cost. But as we refined our approach, I realized the real value wasn't in moving faster—it was in offering more customized, ideal treatments that truly set us apart. The technology became a differentiator rather than a driver."

The Tech-Forward clinician thrives on learning and implementing new systems. They speak at conferences, write for industry publications, and maintain active relationships with equipment manufacturers. Their satisfaction comes from providing patients with treatment options that weren't available even 18 months ago.

Ideal Patient Profile: Tech-savvy professionals, early adopters, patients with complex cases seeking advanced solutions, and those willing to invest in premium care for superior outcomes.

Evolution Pathway: Often begins as traditional practice that gradually incorporates more technology. May transition toward Boutique Experience if the clinician desires more personalized care, or toward Multi-Location Empire if systems become scalable.

2. The Boutique Experience

Marketing Focus: Low Meta, Medium Google, High Web

Premium, highly personalized patient care with exceptional attention to detail. These practices serve fewer patients but command higher fees through superior service and intimate clinician-patient relationships.

Dr. Tracy Li Cheung of Orthodontic Harmony in Briarcliff Manor, New York, exemplifies the boutique model. Nine years ago, she started her practice, then three years later transitioned to a fully concierge model. By eliminating traditional front desk staff and developing streamlined systems, she created a practice that operates just 12 clinical days per month between 9AM and 4PM with a 1.5-hour lunch break—no weekends, early mornings, or evenings.

With over $500,000 in collections per full-time employee and only 10% employee overhead, her fewer team members ensure every patient interaction is intentional and personalized. "We're focused on delivering a bespoke, concierge-level experience without chasing volume. And patients feel the difference."

The Boutique clinician often has artistic sensibilities, values craftsmanship, and derives satisfaction from creating exceptional outcomes for a select patient base.

Ideal Patient Profile: High-income professionals, patients prioritizing quality over cost, individuals seeking cosmetic enhancements, and those who value personal relationships with their healthcare providers.

Evolution Pathway: Often evolves from clinicians who started in higher-volume models but discovered they preferred quality over quantity. May transition toward Lifestyle Practice as personal priorities shift.

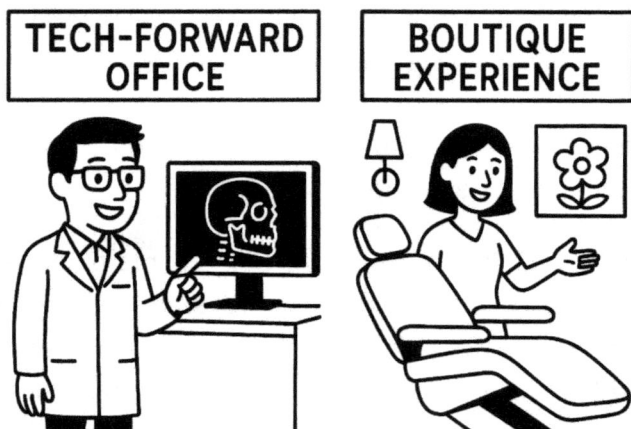

TECH-FORWARD OFFICE

BOUTIQUE EXPERIENCE

3. The High-Volume Clinic

Marketing Focus: High Meta, High Google, High Web

Accessibility, efficiency, and serving large numbers of patients with consistent, quality care. These practices focus on streamlined systems, optimized scheduling, and often accept a wide range of insurance plans.

Dr. Carter Thomas built his orthodontic practice on the principle that everyone deserves excellent care regardless of financial situation. Operating three locations in Mobile, Alabama with his partner Dr. Harvey, his high-volume model features multiple treatment chairs, efficient appointment scheduling, comprehensive insurance acceptance, and systems that allow them to serve thousands of patients while maintaining quality standards.

The High-Volume clinician often has a service-oriented mindset, derives satisfaction from helping large numbers of people, and excels at systematic thinking.

Ideal Patient Profile: Families seeking convenient access, patients prioritizing insurance acceptance, busy professionals needing flexible scheduling, and community members who value efficient, reliable care.

Evolution Pathway: Often begins with clinicians who want to maximize their community impact. May evolve toward Multi-Location Empire through systematization, or transition to Lifestyle Practice as personal priorities change.

4. The Multi-Location Empire

Marketing Focus: High Meta, High Google, High Web

Scalable systems, brand recognition, and leveraged growth across multiple practices. These clinicians focus on building replicable systems, developing leadership teams, and creating practices that operate successfully without their daily presence.

Dr. Greg Efros demonstrates this practice personality type through his systematic expansion from his initial practice to multiple locations across New York's Hudson Valley, including Kingston, Hudson, and Delmar. Through strategic development of protocols, team training programs, and operational systems, he's achieved remarkable growth—

including 37% production increases and $1.7 million in net income benefits—while maintaining his position as a top 1% Invisalign provider nationwide.

Dr. Joseph Mullen represents the evolution pathway to this model. After two years out of residency and associating at two private offices, he just bought his own office in February and is now transitioning and rebranding—building the foundation for systematic growth that could eventually support multiple locations.

The Multi-Location clinician has entrepreneurial instincts, enjoys strategic thinking and team development, and finds satisfaction in building something larger than themselves.

Ideal Patient Profile: Families seeking reliable, consistent care with convenient locations, patients who value established brands and systems, and those requiring comprehensive family dental services.

Evolution Pathway: Usually develops from successful single-location practices that systematize their operations. May incorporate Tech-Forward elements across locations or maintain Boutique Experience standards at scale.

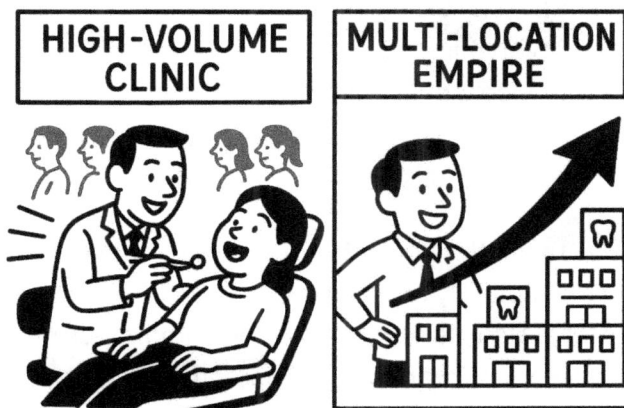

5. The Lifestyle Practice

Marketing Focus: Low Meta, Medium/High Google, High Web

Intentionally designed operations around the clinician's personal priorities. These practices feature compressed schedules, premium pricing, and exceptional work-life integration.

Dr. Brian Rochford exemplifies this evolution beautifully. When he joined his childhood practice in 2017, it was a $2 million traditional operation with paper charts, alginate impressions, and no aligners. Through strategic technology investments and systematic process development, he transformed it into a $5.1 million fully digital practice featuring Invisalign and digital custom braces.

Working just 27 hours per week since going solo in 2022, Dr. Rochford maintains 50% overhead through premium positioning and operational efficiency. His heavy investment in consultants and SOPs (Standard Operating Procedures) for "literally everything" created systems so robust he's now expanding to location #2 with doctor #2, proving that lifestyle practices can be both highly profitable and systematically scalable.

Dr. Emily Taing Watson's transformation provides another powerful example. By redesigning her schedule around family priorities and staff needs, she not only improved her quality of life but also saw dramatic practice growth—from $900K to $3.4 million while working fewer, more focused days.

The lifestyle practice model proves that sustainable success doesn't require constant sacrifice. Another Emily, Dr. Emily Caskey Peppers, who's worked just 8 days per month for 12 years, puts it perfectly: "I'm a huge believer that one of the best things about this career is that we can be focusing on work-life integration throughout our careers, not just toward retirement." Her approach—maintaining a reduced schedule to accommodate her children's needs while her husband teaches public school—demonstrates that lifestyle practices aren't dependent on high-earning spouses but on intentional design and premium positioning.

Dr. Peppers is even planning to take a year off to travel with her family, proving that when you build a practice around your authentic priorities, extraordinary flexibility becomes possible.

Ideal Patient Profile: Patients who value quality over convenience, families seeking long-term clinician relationships, individuals willing to pay premium fees for exceptional care.

Evolution Pathway: Often represents the evolution of clinicians who previously operated higher-volume models but reorganized around personal priorities, or the natural maturation of a startup practice as it finds its sustainable rhythm over time.

6. The Startup Journey

Marketing Focus: Depends on one's desired growth trajectory

New practices or established practices undergoing significant reinvention. These clinicians are in transition, experimenting with different approaches while developing their authentic practice identity.

Dr. Eytan Zarabi perfectly embodies this persona. After graduating in 2023, he bought an office in 2024, but as he describes it, the practice "was very old and run down. It essentially felt like a start-up." Rather than inheriting a functioning model, Dr. Zarabi faces the exciting challenge of building his practice identity from the ground up.

The Startup clinician experiences both excitement and uncertainty as they shape their professional identity. They have the advantage of designing their practice intentionally from the beginning but face the challenges of establishing systems, building patient relationships, and achieving financial stability.

Evolution Pathway: By definition, a transitional persona that develops into one of the other five models as the practice matures and the clinician's preferences become clear.

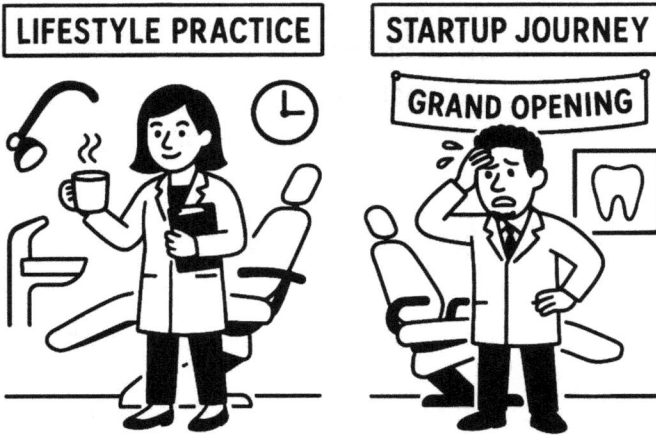

The Marketing Mismatch That's Costing You Everything

Here's a cautionary tale that illustrates a costly mistake we see far too often. This orthodontist—we'll call her Dr. Katherine since understandably, no one wants their name attached to a $47,000 marketing disaster—ran a boutique practice and spent that entire sum on Facebook advertising in one year, targeting families with messaging about "affordable braces for everyone."

The result? Hundreds of leads from parents expecting $99 down payments and monthly plans under $150.

"I was getting tons of calls," she recalls, "but every consultation ended with sticker shock. Parents would see my comprehensive treatment plans and premium materials, then ask if I took Medicaid. I was attracting exactly the wrong patients while my ideal clients—professionals who valued quality and relationship—never saw my ads. Meanwhile, my website looked like every other practice in town, completely failing to communicate the premium experience I actually delivered."

This expensive mistake illustrates a critical truth: **your marketing strategy isn't separate from your practice personality type—it's the external expression of your internal identity.**

When these don't align, you waste money, and worse, you actively repel the patients you most want to serve.

The Evolution Trigger Points

Practice personality types tend to shift at specific life trigger points.

1. The Family Reality Check typically hits between years 5-10, when clinicians realize their demanding schedules are stealing irreplaceable moments with loved ones.

Dr. Jared Lee experienced this during an unprecedented convergence of challenges. In early 2020, as COVID-19 began reshaping dental practice operations, his wife Debi was simultaneously undergoing chemotherapy treatment. The dual crisis forced him to confront how dependent his successful Ventura County practice had become on his constant presence.

"Those early COVID months were unlike anything we'd experienced," Dr. Lee reflects. "Managing practice shutdowns and new safety protocols while being present for Debi during her treatment taught me that our systems needed to be more resilient and less dependent on my constant availability."

Rather than simply surviving the immediate crisis, Dr. Lee used this period to fundamentally reassess his practice model. When the opportunity arose to acquire Hodges Orthodontics, he recognized it as strategic evolution rather than simple expansion. By bringing on Dr. Mullen as an associate and integrating the practices, he created operational redundancy that hadn't existed before.

"The acquisition wasn't about working less—it was about working smarter," he explains. "Now when life requires my attention, whether it's family needs or unexpected circumstances, the practice can continue serving patients at the same high level."

2. The Burnout Breaking Point often occurs around year 15, when clinicians realize they've built practices that require them to be someone they're not.

3. The Legacy Question typically emerges in the final third of careers: "What impact will my practice have beyond my income?"

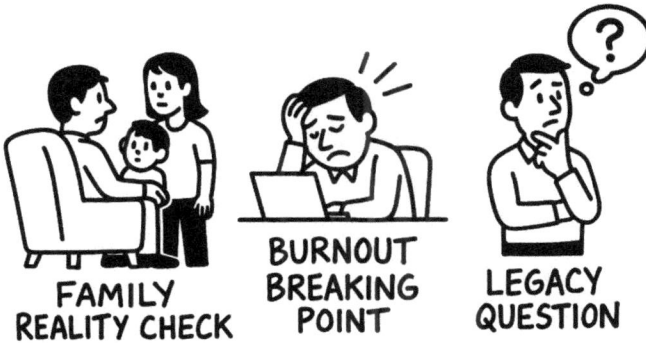

EVOLUTION TRIGGER POINTS

FAMILY REALITY CHECK

BURNOUT BREAKING POINT

LEGACY QUESTION

Your Practice Personality Type Implementation

Don't wait for burnout or family emergencies to force change.

The 5-Minute Personality Type Assessment:

1. **Energy Source:** What aspect of practice energizes you most—learning new technology, building deep patient relationships, solving complex cases efficiently, or creating systematic growth?

2. **Ideal Tuesday:** If you could design your perfect workday without financial constraints, what would it look like?

3. **Success Definition:** When you imagine professional success five years from now, what does it include?

4. **Stress Triggers:** What current practice aspects drain your energy?

5. **Non-Negotiables:** What personal commitments will you never sacrifice for practice demands?

Your answers reveal patterns pointing toward your natural personality type.

The Bottom Line

Your practice personality type is a blueprint for professional fulfillment that honors both your capabilities and your humanity.

The practice of your dreams isn't somewhere out there waiting to be discovered. It's waiting to be created through the deliberate alignment of who you are with how you choose to serve your patients and structure your professional life.

Most clinicians spend more time planning their vacations than designing their practice identity. Then they wonder why Monday mornings feel like punishment instead of possibility.

Stop building someone else's practice. Start building yours.

The question isn't whether you can afford to align your practice with your authentic personality type.

The question is: how much longer can you afford not to?

Key Takeaways

- Misalignment between who you are and your practice personality is a primary cause of burnout.

- There are six proven practice personality types—each with its own strengths, patient fit, and marketing approach.

- Your practice personality type is not static; it evolves with your life stage and priorities.

- Marketing is effective only when it matches your practice type; misalignment wastes time and money.

- Defining your type lets you build with intention instead of defaulting to someone else's model.

Next Steps

Start creating alignment between you and your practice now.

Take the 5-Minute Personality Type Assessment: Define your energy sources, stress triggers, and non-negotiables.

Evaluate alignment: Does your current practice model reflect your authentic self, or one you inherited?

Choose one adjustment: Start with one area—scheduling, staffing, or marketing—that will bring your practice closer to your true type.

Defining your practice personality is a huge step towards practice freedom. The real test is whether your team can live it out every day. If they don't understand or embody your vision, your practice model remains just an idea.

That's why leadership and culture matter so much. Your practice can only grow as far as your team grows. In the next chapter, we'll explore how to build a culture that empowers your team, amplifies your practice personality, and frees you to focus on what matters most.

Chapter 5: Team Culture and Leadership

By: Dr. Kyle Fagala

Dr. Rebecca sat at her desk, staring at the calendar, as the afternoon sun cut through the blinds. Three weeks until her daughter's graduation—and not a single gap in her schedule. She had missed the science fair last month, and now this milestone was in jeopardy as well. Her team was strong, capable, and eager to take on more responsibility, yet she carried the weight of every task herself. Insurance forms, supply orders, even approving the smallest decisions— everything flowed back to her. The result was exhaustion, missed family moments, and a practice that felt like it owned her, rather than the other way around.

Your team holds the keys to your freedom. Leadership in practice isn't about doing everything yourself—it's about empowering others to lead with you. When you build systems of trust, training, and responsibility, you unlock the full potential of your team and create a practice that thrives even when you're not in the building.

The practice model and the relationships you want to build depend on a team that's aligned with your vision. And your team can't align if you never let them lead. That's why the next step is creating a culture where your people are empowered to take ownership, freeing you to focus on the work only you can do.

You'll discover how leadership is less about control and more about empowerment, how culture can transform your team into true partners, and why letting go strategically makes your practice stronger. You'll understand how to build systems that multiply your impact instead of draining your energy.

You Are Your Own Jailor

Let's be honest—many clinicians find themselves trapped in a prison of their own making.

You've built a thriving practice that now demands your constant presence, leaving little room for family, hobbies, or even a simple vacation without your phone buzzing every few minutes.

This reality exists because too many healthcare leaders believe only they can perform the crucial functions that keep their practices running.

It's not just incorrect—it's unsustainable.

The irony is striking. You entered your profession to help others and create a fulfilling life, yet now find yourself working 60-hour weeks, handling tasks any properly trained team member could manage. Your expertise is being diluted across administrative duties, routine procedures, and managerial firefighting that pulls you away from your highest value work.

Meanwhile, your team watches from the sidelines, capabilities untapped, waiting for permission to truly contribute.

This chapter confronts a fundamental truth: your practice will never outgrow your ability to delegate.

Without strategic empowerment of your team, you've created a demanding dependence that follows you everywhere.

The most successful practice owners aren't those who do everything themselves—they're the ones who systematically train others to execute with excellence, creating a culture that thrives whether they're in the building or not.

The Liberation of Leadership

True leadership in a healthcare practice is **about systematically distributing control.**

When you empower your team through training, clear systems, and gradually increasing responsibility, you create something revolutionary: a practice that serves both your patients and your life.

The clinicians who achieve this balance understand that building team capability is **the only real path to sustainability**.

That's because what your team members are looking for is mastery, autonomy, and purpose. When you build a culture that provides these elements, you transform ordinary employees into practice champions who take ownership, solve problems independently, and maintain standards even in your absence.

But here's what you've got to remember: this transformation requires intentional leadership and systems designed for continuous development.

Another Milestone Missed?

That afternoon, the intercom buzzed: another patient was ready, and another assistant was out sick. Dr. Rebecca's shoulders slumped as she reached for the stack of insurance forms Jack, her office manager, had left. He knew the business inside and out—yet she still insisted on signing off on every detail. Melissa, her hygienist, had recently completed advanced training and was thriving in her role. Rebecca could see her anticipating patient needs with precision, building trust effortlessly. But instead of empowering Melissa and Jack to lead more, Rebecca double-checked their work, creating bottlenecks that drained her energy.

She picked up her daughter's graduation invitation again, the gold lettering glinting in the light. She thought of her own father, who had once closed his shop for a day to be at her graduation. He had trusted his assistant manager to keep things running, and not only had the shop survived—it had thrived with a new idea that boosted sales. Rebecca realized she was holding her team back the same way she was holding herself back. The problem wasn't their capability—it was her unwillingness to let go.

The turning point came as she looked through the window at Melissa preparing the operatory, her confidence evident. If her team could manage the practice in small moments, why not in larger ways? Rebecca knew then that empowering her staff wasn't about abdicating responsibility—it was about giving them the chance to lead, so she could show up where she mattered most: for her patients, her practice vision, and her family.

You Are the Bus Driver:
The Energy You Bring Changes Everything

In Jon Gordon's powerful book The Energy Bus, he shares a fundamental truth that every orthodontist and dentist must understand: **you are the bus driver of your practice.**

There are only two ways to influence human behavior: you can manipulate it, or you can inspire it. This principle transforms how we think about team leadership in healthcare practices. As the leader, you provide the most important and essential energy to the mix. Your energy—positive or negative—sets the tone for everything that happens in your practice, and that inspiration makes all the difference.

The Energy Bus teaches us that positive people and positive teams create positive results.

Think about it: your team feeds off your energy every single day. When you walk into the practice feeling stressed, overwhelmed, or defeated, that energy spreads like wildfire. But when you arrive with purpose, optimism, and clarity about your "why," something magical happens—your team rises to meet that standard.

The key insight from The Energy Bus is understanding that enthusiasm is contagious.

Over thousands of centuries, humans have developed the ability to understand emotions from afar through body language and energy. Studies show our heart has its own electromagnetic field, and the waves it sends can be sensed by others, even if they're up to ten feet away.

The Energy Formula: E + P = O

Jon Gordon shares a powerful formula: Energy plus Perception equals Outcome (E + P = O). When your perception is positive, you'll create positive outcomes. As the practice leader, your perception of challenges, opportunities, and your team's capabilities directly influences the results you achieve.

But here's the crucial part: **once you identify negative energy on your bus, you must get it off immediately.**

This might be the most difficult yet important decision you'll make as a leader. Toxic team members don't just affect productivity—they poison the culture and drain the positive energy from everyone around them.

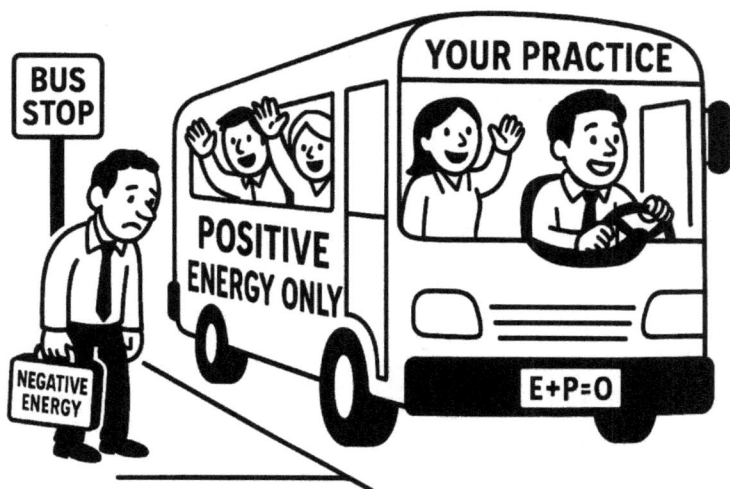

Choosing Your Passengers Wisely

Great companies don't hire skilled people and motivate them—they hire already motivated people and inspire them.

This means hiring for attitude and cultural fit first, then training for skills. A positive, eager team member who believes in your practice's mission will always outperform a technically skilled person who brings negative energy to your environment.

When building your team, ask yourself: Would I want to be on a long bus trip with this person? Do they bring energy that lifts others up, or do they drain the room? Your practice culture is too important to compromise on this principle.

The Disney Standard:
Creating Magic Through Culture

Speaking at a continuing education event in Kansas City, I was making a lighthearted joke about Snow White and how impossible it would be to show up and be that cheerful every single day. A table nearby started snickering, so I asked what was going on. It turned out one of the team members had actually worked as Snow White at Disney for a couple of years.

"How did you manage to be so positive and cheerful every day?" I asked her.

Her answer revolutionized how I think about team culture. She explained that Disney has **"Princess School"** every single morning before the characters head out into the park. They do calisthenics, practice their autographs, and most importantly, they're reminded of Disney's core values.

Disney's Four Keys have guided their legendary service for more than 60 years: Safety, Courtesy, Show, and Efficiency. In 2021, they added a fifth key: Inclusion. These values are lived and breathed by every Cast Member, every single day.

Making the Mundane Magical

Think about what Disney accomplishes: they take the experience of standing in long lines, spending too much money, eating mediocre food, and riding decent rides, and somehow transform it into an exceptional, magical experience that people plan years in advance and pay premium prices to enjoy.

This is a masterful example of team culture in action.

How does this apply to your practice? We all bring "stuff" to work each day—stress and anxiety over relationships, finances, personal challenges. But Disney's approach teaches us that we must choose to leave that stuff in the car and commit to being our best selves for the benefit of our teams and patients.

Your Morning "Princess School"

Consider implementing your own version of Princess School through daily morning huddles. Patrick Lencioni's Death by Meeting shows us that brief, daily check-ins can be incredibly powerful when done correctly. These 5-10 minute standing meetings ensure nothing falls through the cracks and people don't step on each other's toes.

During these huddles:

- Review the day's schedule and any special patient needs
- Address any immediate operational issues
- Reinforce your practice values and "why"
- Celebrate wins from the previous day
- Set the positive energy tone for the day ahead

To embed this in people's routines, keep the meetings at the same time and location, and make sure you don't cancel even if only two team members are in the office on a given day.

Start with Why:
The Foundation of Practice Culture

Simon Sinek's groundbreaking concept teaches us that **people don't buy what you do—they buy why you do it.**

The most successful leaders and organizations think, act, and communicate from the inside out, starting with their core purpose, cause, or belief.

The Golden Circle in Practice

The Golden Circle consists of three levels: Why (your core purpose), How (your unique processes and values), and What (your tangible services and results). Most practices communicate from the outside in, starting with "What," but inspiring leaders begin with "Why."

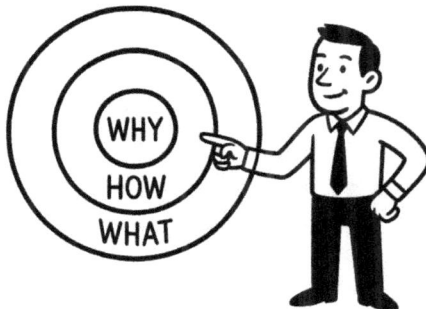

For orthodontists and dentists, this means:

> **WHY:** Why do you exist beyond making money? Perhaps it's to boost confidence, improve health, or transform lives through beautiful smiles.

> **HOW:** What makes your approach unique? Maybe it's your advanced technology, personalized care, or family-focused environment.

> **WHAT:** What services do you provide? Invisalign, traditional braces, cosmetic dentistry, implants, etc.

Building a Why-Driven Culture

When employees belong and understand the "why," they will guarantee your success.

There's a mindset shift that comes with this transformation. Instead of working hard and looking for innovative solutions just for you, they'll do it for themselves. The goal is to hire those who are passionate about your "Why," your purpose, cause, or belief, and who have the attitude that fits your culture.

When your team understands and believes in your practice's deeper purpose, they stop thinking of patients as appointments and start seeing them as lives to transform. They stop viewing problems as interruptions and start seeing them as opportunities to live out your shared mission.

The Power of Empowering Leadership

Leadership in healthcare practices often follows traditional hierarchical models. The clinician leads, and staff follows. This approach can work effectively in many circumstances, especially during critical clinical moments when quick decisions are essential.

However, it also creates a bottleneck where every decision, approval, and process must filter through a single person— you.

Think of your practice as an orchestra. Traditional leadership casts you as both conductor and first violin. You're setting the tempo while simultaneously trying to play your part perfectly. It's exhausting and ultimately unsustainable.

Empowering leadership styles flip this dynamic.

By training team members to take ownership of specific areas, you multiply your effectiveness. Research consistently shows that practices with distributed leadership experience less burnout among clinicians while maintaining or improving quality metrics.

This approach helps you strategically reallocate your respon-sibilities to create a more resilient organization, while still maintaining the integrity of your role.

The Transition Challenge

The transition isn't always smooth. Many clinicians struggle with letting go, fearing quality will suffer or believing no one else can perform tasks to their standards. This perfectionistic thinking creates a self-fulfilling prophecy: by never allowing team members to develop skills, they never become proficient enough to meet your standards.

Successful practice leaders understand that different situations call for different leadership approaches:

- **During training:** A more directive style may be appropriate
- **As team members develop:** A coaching approach helps them grow
- **Eventually:** A delegative style where you provide resources and support while team members execute independently

The Payoff

The payoff for this transition is substantial. Practitioners who embrace empowering leadership report:

- More time for focused clinical work
- Greater work-life balance
- Increased job satisfaction

- Higher team engagement
- Lower turnover
- More innovation
- Better patient experience

Most importantly, empowering leadership requires trusting your team.

This trust must be genuine and visible. When you demonstrate that you believe in your team's capabilities, they rise to meet your expectations. The practice transforms from being clinician-dependent to team-driven, creating space for everyone to contribute their best work.

Real-Time Communication: The Moment-of-Truth Principle

One critical aspect of building strong team culture often gets overlooked: **the importance of addressing issues in the moment.**

You don't need to embarrass your team in front of patients, but you should be willing to address concerns right then and there. Waiting days, weeks, or months to tell someone about an issue elevates the emotions and makes it feel like a betrayal or "knife in the back" rather than simply pulling off a band-aid.

When you see something that needs correction:

1. Wait for an appropriate private moment
2. Address it calmly and specifically
3. Focus on the behavior, not the person
4. Provide clear expectations going forward
5. Follow up to ensure understanding

This approach builds trust because team members know where they stand. They appreciate the immediate feedback rather than wondering if you're keeping a mental list of their mistakes.

Building a Learning Culture

Creating systems for continuous team development takes **intentional design and consistent implementation.**

Practices that excel at team development share common characteristics: they budget time and resources specifically for training, they recognize and reward growth, and they view skill development as a strategic advantage rather than an expense.

What does this look like in practice?

- Schedule regular "lunch and learn" sessions where team members can share knowledge

- Implement a continuing education allowance that team members can direct toward their professional interests
- Create a skills matrix that clearly outlines growth pathways within your organization

These structured approaches signal to your team that development matters.

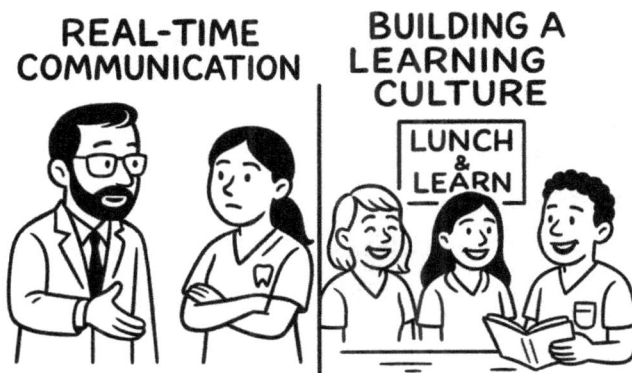

REAL-TIME COMMUNICATION

BUILDING A LEARNING CULTURE

LUNCH & LEARN

The Cost of Not Developing Your Team

How many talented team members have you lost because they couldn't see a future at your practice?

The cost of turnover is staggering—not just financially, but in lost institutional knowledge, disrupted patient relationships, and team morale. By contrast, practices with robust development systems often report retention rates 40% higher than industry averages.

Clinical skills are only one part of team development. Technical training provides one essential element, but interpersonal skills, leadership capabilities, and cultural fit are equally important for total success.

Consider the ripple effect of investment in your team.

When one team member learns a new skill, they often share it informally with colleagues. This organic knowledge transfer multiplies your initial investment. Furthermore, team members who feel invested in become investors themselves—contributing ideas, effort, and loyalty beyond what's required in their job descriptions.

Team members stay where they're growing. They remain engaged when they can see their progress. They commit to organizations that commit to them.

Relationship Expiration Dates and Hiring Philosophy

Here's a hard truth about team culture: **all relationships have an expiration date.**

Once a relationship expires—when a team member is no longer growing, contributing, or aligned with your culture—you must be willing to fire fast. Keeping the wrong people on your team too long can hurt productivity, sure—but on a deeper level it can damage the morale of your good team members who end up carrying extra weight.

The flip side is equally important: hire slow.

Take time to really understand who you're bringing onto your team:

- Check references thoroughly
- Do working interviews
- Assess cultural fit as much as technical skills

Remember: you want to hire people who are already motivated and passionate about your "why," then inspire them rather than trying to motivate skilled people who don't share your values.

The ECO Framework:
Building a Self-Sustaining Culture

Practitioners who build dependence on their constant presence create a fragile system that risks crumbling during vacation, illness, or family emergencies. The alternative—a resilient practice culture—provides both professional longevity and personal freedom.

Think of your practice culture as a flywheel. Initially, it requires significant energy to start turning. You must push consistently, establishing clear expectations, systems, and values. But once momentum builds, the flywheel keeps spinning with much less effort.

A self-sustaining culture operates on this principle—your initial investment in building the right environment pays dividends long after your active involvement decreases.

The ECO Framework Components

The ECO Framework provides a structured approach to building a self-sustaining practice culture. This model integrates three essential elements that work together to create an environment where team members thrive and the practice operates effectively regardless of the doctor's presence.

E = Empowerment: Beyond Delegation

Empowerment forms the foundation of the ECO Framework. Unlike simple delegation, which merely assigns tasks, true empowerment transfers both responsibility and authority. This distinction is crucial.

When team members are empowered, they make decisions, solve problems, and take initiative within clearly defined boundaries.

Characteristics of effective empowerment include:

- **Clarity of scope:** Team members understand exactly what falls within their authority

- **Training for competence:** Skills are developed before responsibility is transferred

- **Resources for success:** Access to tools, information, and support needed to succeed

- **Psychological safety:** Freedom to make occasional mistakes without fear of punishment

- **Graduated autonomy:** Authority increases as team members demonstrate capability

Empowerment requires clinicians to move beyond the "I'll just do it myself" mentality that often feels efficient in the short term but creates bottlenecks and dependency in the long run.

C = Communication: Creating Alignment

The second element of the ECO Framework is communication. Effective communication creates alignment around values, expectations, and processes that guide decision-making when you're not present. **It's the invisible infrastructure that supports team autonomy while maintaining consistency.**

Key components of communication within this framework include:

- **Values clarification:** Explicitly defining what matters most in your practice

- **Decision guidelines:** Clear criteria for making choices that align with practice values

- **Regular huddles:** Brief team meetings to address emerging issues and celebrate wins
- **Feedback loops:** Structured processes for continuous improvement
- **Transparent information sharing:** Access to relevant data for informed decision-making

Communication must flow in multiple directions—not just from clinician to team, but between team members and from team to clinician.

O = Ownership: Cultivating Investment

The final element of the ECO Framework is ownership— the psychological and emotional investment team members have in the practice's success. **When team members feel ownership, they treat the practice as their own, making decisions that consider long-term success rather than just immediate convenience.**

Strategies for developing ownership include:

- **Shared vision:** Involving the team in defining future goals

- **Recognition systems:** Acknowledging contributions visibly and consistently

- **Growth opportunities:** Creating pathways for advancement within the practice

- **Financial alignment:** Bonus structures that connect individual success to practice success

- **Decision participation:** Including team members in relevant strategic discussions

Ownership transforms the fundamental relationship between team members and the practice. Instead of working "for" the practice, they begin working "as" the practice.

Dynamic Interactions Within the Framework

The power of the ECO Framework lies not just in its individual components but in how they interact:

- Empowerment without communication creates confusion

- Communication without ownership results in compliance rather than commitment

- Ownership without empowerment leads to frustration

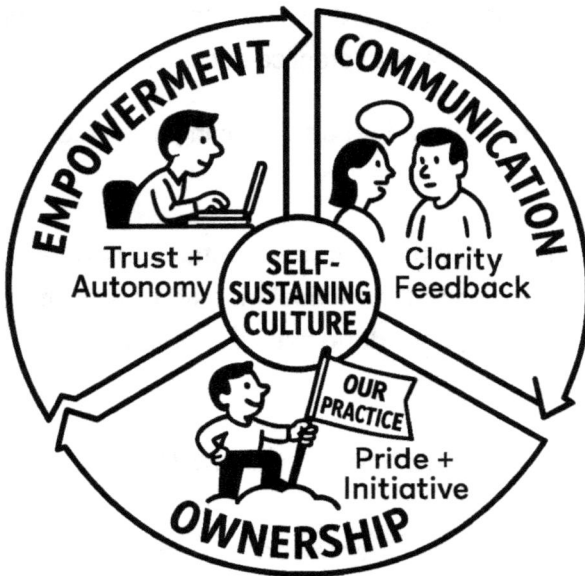

When properly integrated, these elements create positive reinforcement cycles. Empowerment demonstrated through delegated authority builds trust. Communication clarifies expectations and provides feedback. Ownership motivates continuous improvement and initiative.

Together, they form a self-reinforcing system that becomes increasingly stable over time.

Measuring Success

How do you know if your culture-building efforts are working? Look for these indicators:

- Problems are increasingly solved without your intervention
- Team members initiate improvements without prompting
- Quality metrics remain stable during your absence
- Patients speak positively about their interactions with your entire team
- Team turnover decreases while engagement increases

These signs indicate your practice is developing the resilience that comes from shared ownership and distributed leadership. **The culture is becoming self-sustaining—capable of maintaining excellence regardless of your presence.**

The Leadership Paradox Resolved

When you empower your team through intentional leadership, something remarkable happens. The daily pressures that once fell squarely on your shoulders become distributed across capable hands that you've carefully trained and developed.

Remember that culture isn't created by accident. The systems you implement for continuous team development directly impact both your staff retention and your personal freedom. When team members see clear paths for growth, they invest more deeply in your practice's success.

Perhaps most importantly, the practice that can function effectively without your constant oversight is the one that gives you the greatest gift: **choice**.

Choice to be present for your family. Choice to pursue other interests. Choice to expand your practice or simply to enjoy the fruits of the one you've built.

The Virtuous Cycle

This approach creates a virtuous cycle:

- As your team grows more competent, you become less burdened
- As you become less burdened, you have more energy to invest in strategic leadership
- Your practice becomes not just a place of service but a living expression of your values

The paradox resolves itself when you realize that holding on tightly to every aspect of your practice actually weakens it.

By letting go—strategically and systematically—you build something far stronger than you could by maintaining control.

Key Takeaways

- Your practice will never outgrow your ability to delegate.

- Empowering your team requires trust, systems, and consistent leadership.

- Culture is shaped by your energy and reinforced on a daily basis.

- Positive culture multiplies patient trust, staff loyalty, and your freedom.

- Leadership is not about doing more—it's about building others to do more with you.

Next Steps

You don't have to overhaul everything at once. Start small and build momentum:

Choose one task to delegate – Hand off something you currently do that a team member could own with the right training.

Run a daily 5-minute huddle – Align energy, review the schedule, and reinforce your practice values.

Empower one team member – Identify someone ready to grow, give them added responsibility, and support them as they step up.

Your culture, that alignment and energy, is not just for your team and patients; it's the very thing you're marketing. When your practice reflects your authentic self and your team's strengths, your marketing becomes more than promotion; it becomes an invitation. And when you pair that foundation with the right marketing strategies, you don't just attract more patients—you attract the right patients, the ones who energize you, sustain your team, and allow your practice to become exactly what you envisioned.

That's the power of marketing built on a strong foundation. And that's where we turn next.

Section IV: Practice Growth & Operations

Discover:

Chapter 6 – Marketing – Creating New Leads: Why authentic marketing built on your culture attracts the right patients for your practice.

Chapter 7 – The New Patient Journey: How designing the right patient experience supports your vision and builds loyalty.

Chapter 8 – Treatment Coordination and Sales: How masterful treatment coordination converts the right leads into long-term patient advocates.

Chapter 9 – Clinical Implementation Excellence: How systems, protocols, and empowered teams deliver consistent outcomes while freeing you from micromanagement.

Chapter 6: Marketing – Creating New Leads

By: Luke Infinger

Technology: Your Secret Weapon Against Practice Burnout

Dr. Lauren had just returned from a seminar, fired up by the latest technology she'd seen at the trade show. A marketing company had sold her on a tool "guaranteed" to flood her practice with new patients. She signed the contract on the spot.

Back at the office, her staff exchanged wary glances. Here we go again, they thought. *Another bright, shiny object.* The software promised growth, but no one really understood how it worked, how it would fit into their daily systems, or what training they'd receive. Within weeks, the excitement had faded, the tool was underused, and frustration replaced the initial spark.

That's the trap. Too many doctors see technology or marketing as a magic bullet. They buy the tool, flip the switch, and expect instant results. However, the real power lies not in the technology itself. It's in how you implement it, how you train your team to embrace it, and how you align it with the culture and systems of your practice.

Marketing only works when it builds on the foundation you've already created. The strengths of your team, the systems you've put in place, and the personality of your practice form the soil. Technology and marketing are the tools that help it grow. When they're aligned with who you are and how your practice runs, they don't just bring in leads—they bring in the right patients, the ones who make your practice more profitable, more sustainable, and more fulfilling.

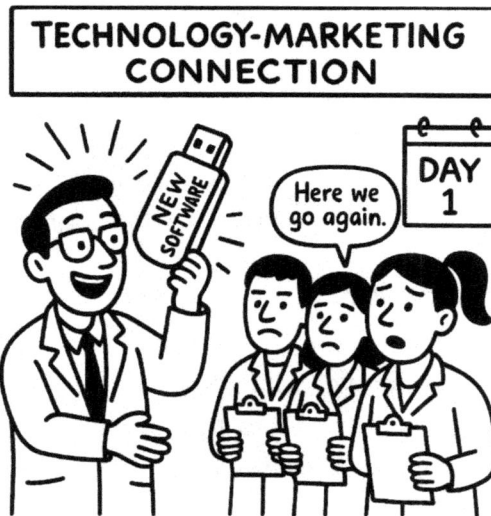

Technology only works when your team buys in. And your team only buys in when you position it properly— showing how it makes their lives easier, saves them time, helps them earn more (especially if bonuses are tied to growth), and improves the care experience for patients.

If you can also replace three or four clunky tools with one streamlined platform? That's a win everyone can feel.

The modern practice faces a fundamental paradox: the very systems designed to help you serve patients often become the barriers that exhaust you. Electronic health records, scheduling software, patient management platforms, etc. These can either liberate your practice or chain it to inefficiency. The difference is how deliberately you align the technology with your practice's vision, values, and workflows.

Too many clinicians overlook the hidden costs of outdated systems. That clunky scheduling process wastes time, costs trust, frustrates staff, and pushes patients away. That glitchy patient management system crashes and eats morale. Those little inefficiencies pile up, day after day, fueling the very burnout you're trying to avoid.

But when technology is chosen thoughtfully and implemented strategically, it makes your practice better for everyone.

Online scheduling gives patients autonomy. Automated follow-ups show them you care even when they're not in the chair. Educational content empowers them to make smarter decisions about their care. Patients notice. They appreciate it. And they stay loyal.

This chapter explores how to stop chasing "magic bullet" software and start making strategic technology investments that support your marketing and your mission. You'll learn how to attract more of your ideal patients—the ones who energize rather than drain you—by aligning your systems, messaging, and team around a clear vision.

We'll break down three essential marketing strategies that sit on top of a solid technology foundation. You'll see how targeted outreach attracts the right patients, how to craft a value proposition that actually connects with your community, and why filtering for fit is just as important as filling your schedule.

The practices thriving in today's healthcare landscape aren't the ones with the biggest budgets or flashiest toys. They're the ones that integrate technology and marketing into a cohesive system that serves the team, delights the patient, and keeps the doctor (you) sane.

Because when your systems actually work, marketing stops feeling like a promotion and starts feeling like a connection.

The Marketing Mindset Shift

Before We Talk Strategy, Let's Talk Mindset

Let's be honest. For many clinicians, the word marketing feels uncomfortable. Maybe even a little dirty. You didn't become a doctor to "sell" people. You became a doctor to help them.

But here's the truth: good marketing is helping people.

The problem is that most practices position themselves the wrong way. They lead with themselves: their credentials, their technology, their beautiful office. Then they wonder why patients don't connect.

People don't care about you. Not yet.

They care about their pain, their frustration, their problems. They want to know you understand what they're going through and that you can fix it. That's where your message needs to start—with them.

What do they feel walking into your practice?

What's keeping them up at night?

What's the emotional weight of their problem?

Address that first. Only then do you earn the right to tell them why you're the doctor to solve it. Your credibility, your technology, and your service still matter. But sequence matters more.

Effective marketing isn't about convincing people to buy something they don't need. It's about showing the right people you understand them and can help. When your message reflects what your patients actually care about, you attract the right ones and naturally filter out the wrong ones. That alignment between your marketing, your values, and your clinical reality creates fulfilling professional relationships that energize you instead of draining you.

Dr. Jason sat in his office, staring at his phone. The last email he'd sent to his marketing rep still sat unanswered, though it had only been two hours. Outside his window, a steady drizzle coated the parking lot. The gray sky matched his mood.

It had been 45 days since he signed on with the new marketing company his friend Mark had recommended. The pitch had been impressive, the team seemed sharp, and their ideas sounded like exactly what his practice needed. But here he was, six weeks later, and the number of new patient exams hadn't really changed.

Frustrated, he scrolled to Mark's contact and hit call.

"Hey man," Jason said when Mark picked up. "Quick question about that marketing company you told me about."

"Yeah," Mark replied. "What's going on?"

Jason sighed. "Honestly? I'm not seeing it. It's been six weeks, and nothing's really improved. I thought this was supposed to fix my marketing."

There was a pause, then Mark chuckled. "You sound exactly like I did at first. Let me save you some time. It took me eight months before things really snowballed."

Jason frowned. "Eight months? Seriously?"

"Seriously," Mark said. "And you know why? Because I stopped treating them like a vendor and started treating them like a partner."

Jason leaned back. "What do you mean?"

"I mean," Mark continued, "you can't just write the check and wait for magic. This isn't a slot machine where you pull the handle and win overnight. It's more like real estate—you've got to put in the work, stay involved, and give it time to appreciate."

Jason stayed quiet, listening.

"When I started giving them real-time feedback— what kinds of calls were coming in, what patients were saying, where we were losing people—they adjusted. When I worked with my team to make sure operations could actually handle the leads, everything started compounding. And now it runs like a machine."

The words stuck with him. Compounding. Appreciating. Partnering.

He realized he'd been treating his marketing investment like it was someone else's job. Write a check, walk away, wait for results.

But that wasn't business ownership. That was wishful thinking.

Jason hung up and sat in silence for a moment, watching cars pull in and out of the lot below. The world didn't reward people who planted seeds and walked away expecting a harvest the next day. It rewarded those who stayed in the dirt, kept watering, and let the roots take hold.

That was the difference between hiring a vendor and building a partnership.

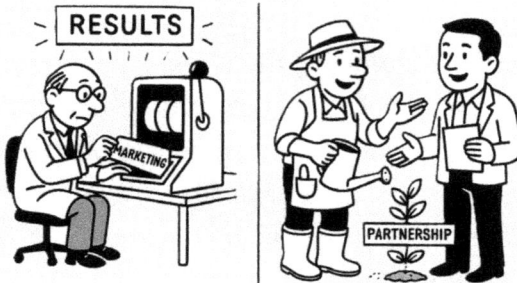

One was just spending money. The other was building something that could actually grow.

Finding Your Target: Precision in Patient Acquisition

Marketing isn't about casting the widest net. It is about showing up where your patients already are, on their phones, and connecting with them in a way that resonates.

Here's what most practices overlook: it is not only about attracting patients who already know they need treatment. Many of your best patients are the ones who have not yet realized that they or their child could benefit from it. That mom scrolling Instagram at 10 p.m. has no idea the AAO recommends an orthodontic evaluation by age seven until your ad tells her. That dad on Google searching "why is my son grinding his teeth at night" doesn't know what options are out there until your search campaign shows up with answers.

That's the power of modern marketing technology. It doesn't just reach people who are looking. It helps people who should be looking find you.

Too many doctors overcomplicate targeting. They spend hours obsessing over data and demographics when the platforms already know more than you ever could. Meta and Google have the data. Your only job is to craft the right message— the right copy—that speaks to your ideal patient's needs, frustrations, and emotions.

On Facebook and Instagram, the algorithm will find the right people if your creative is compelling. On Google, the right keywords and ad structure surface your practice to the ones actively searching now.

Forget generic messaging like "We treat everyone with care." That doesn't connect. Instead, write to a specific audience with a specific outcome. **"We help moms stay ahead of their child's orthodontic needs with early evaluations that save time, money, and hassle." Or: "We help adults finally feel confident in their smile—without anyone noticing they're in treatment."**

That level of specificity cuts through the noise.

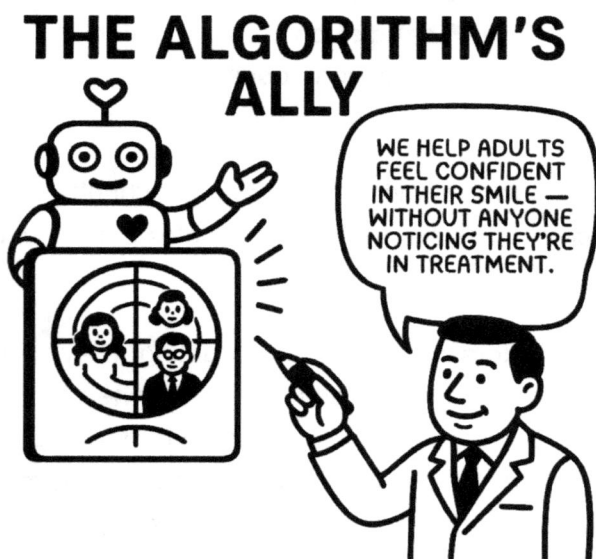

Many clinicians hesitate to narrow their focus, worried they'll turn people away. But broad messaging attracts no one. Specific messaging attracts the right ones.

Technology enables you to amplify that message at scale—without guessing. Social platforms, search engines, and digital ads already know who's most likely to engage. When your creative is dialed in and your team is ready to convert interest into appointments, your marketing becomes a machine.

Marketing is no longer just about finding the right patients who already know they need you. It's about creating awareness, sparking interest, and guiding people toward care they didn't even realize was possible.

That's the real advantage of aligning your marketing with modern technology. It lets you meet patients where they are, show them what's possible, and invite them into a better future with your practice.

Communicating Your Difference: Creating Value That Matters

In orthodontics and dentistry today, patients have more options than ever. They're still comparing you to the doctor across town, but they're also weighing you against virtual consults, mail-order aligners, and big-box corporate practices.

So, why should they choose you?

The answer is simple—yet often overlooked. It's your *unique value proposition* (UVP): the clear, specific, meaningful reason a patient should trust you with their care instead of going elsewhere.

And here's the truth: your UVP isn't about what you say you offer. It's about what your patients feel you deliver.

Your UVP sits at the intersection of three questions:

- What do you and your team do exceptionally well?

- What do your ideal patients care about most?

- How are you different from the alternatives they're already considering?

Here's what it's not: a clever tagline, a vague promise of "quality care," or "we treat everyone like family." Those things are forgettable.

Here's what it could be:

- "We help busy professionals transform their smile discreetly with clear aligners—without disrupting their lifestyle."

- "We help anxious kids feel confident in the chair, and confident in their smile, starting at age 7."

- "We help adults who thought it was too late finally get the healthy, beautiful smile they deserve."

Your UVP doesn't need to appeal to everyone. It shouldn't. Like the best restaurants with a tight menu, you're not trying to be everything to everyone. You're perfecting a specific experience that speaks directly to the people you want to serve most.

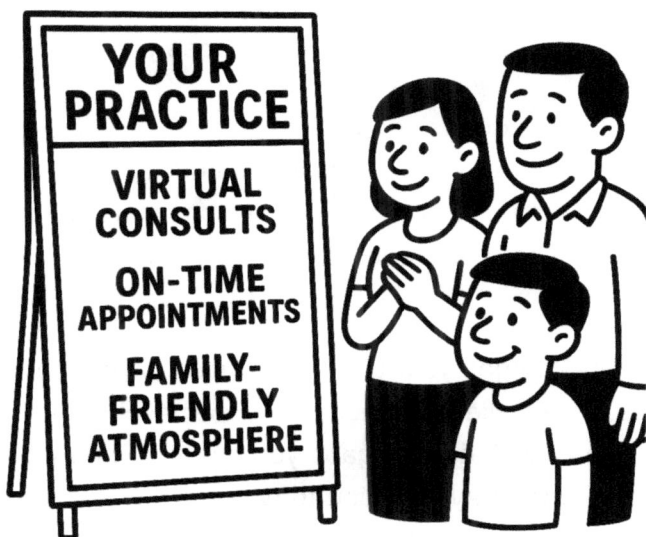

Too many practices try to compete on "we care" and "we're friendly." Those aren't differentiators—they're the price of admission. **Your UVP should show patients something they can't get from a corporate chain or a DIY app. Something that speaks to their priorities, their emotions, and their vision of what's possible.**

Once you define it, you need to communicate it. Everywhere.

- Your website should clearly spell it out, supported by testimonials and before-and-afters.

- Your ads should echo it in words and images patients actually relate to.

- Your social posts should reinforce it with real stories, not stock slogans.

- Your team should be able to say it out loud when a patient asks: "Why should I choose you?"

The best UVPs go beyond clinical outcomes. They touch the whole experience. Do you make scheduling seamless? Do you run on time? Do you offer virtual consultations or flexible payment options? Do patients walk out feeling understood and valued?

Finally, don't forget: your UVP isn't static. As your community evolves, your patients' needs and expectations change too. Keep listening. Watch for gaps you can fill. Survey patients. Talk to parents. Pay attention to what frustrates them about other providers, and solve it better.

Patients don't just need a dentist or an orthodontist. They need a reason to choose *you*.

So what's your reason? And more importantly—are you saying it clearly, consistently, and confidently enough that your patients believe it?

The Right Fit: Marketing for Mutual Satisfaction

At times, filling your schedule can feel hard—especially in a competitive market or when you're still building momentum. But the truth is, ***anyone* can fill a schedule if they lower their standards enough**. Big discounts, giveaways, and generic ads can generate a lot of busy work.

What actually transforms your practice—and your daily experience as a clinician—is filling your schedule with the *right* patients. People who can actually say, yes!

When your chairs are full of patients who value your expertise, trust your process, and are committed to their care, your satisfaction skyrockets.

But we've all experienced the opposite. The mismatched patient who expects miracles overnight. The parent who questions every decision but never follows through. The adult who disappears halfway through treatment. Those mismatches drain energy, strain the team, and hurt outcomes.

That's why your marketing and follow-up process should do more than just generate leads. It should filter out those who aren't a fit to come in and move forward. At the same time, **it should nurture those who aren't ready today but could be in the future**—keeping your practice top of mind until the timing is right.

Think of your marketing as matchmaking. Just as dating apps don't just connect random people, your ads, messaging, and creative should attract the kind of patients who thrive under your care—and quietly discourage those who won't.

This starts with clarity. Your website, ads, and social posts should clearly explain how you work, what you expect from patients, and what they can expect from you. Are you all about early intervention? Do you prioritize aesthetics and discreet options for busy adults? Are you committed to a specific kind of experience—warm, personal, family-centered? Say so.

When you communicate your philosophy upfront, patients start to self-select. That mom who sees herself in your messaging will call. That adult who resonates with your patient stories will book. Everyone else may move on—and that's exactly what you want.

Real examples help. Video testimonials from patients who embody your ideal relationships are some of the most effective tools you can use. Let prospective patients hear what it's like to work with you from someone who already has.

It's also about follow-through. Once they're in the door, every touchpoint should reinforce the values you promised in your marketing. From how your team answers the phone to how easy scheduling is to how treatment is explained—patients should feel like they made the right choice at every step.

Think of it like a restaurant. The menu, decor, service, and price point all attract the right diners and set expectations. If someone walks into a fine-dining restaurant expecting fast food, no one's happy. Same with your practice.

When you get this right, everything gets easier. Patients show up. They follow through. They pay on time. They tell their friends. And you and your team can focus on what you do best instead of chasing no-shows and calming frustrated parents.

Which leaves the real payoff: a practice that feels better to run.

Marketing done right isn't just about getting more patients. It's about getting the *right* ones. The ones who make your work more rewarding and your outcomes more predictable.

And that's not just good for business. That's good for you.

The Technology-Marketing Connection

Targeted strategies, clear value propositions, and attracting the right patients all rely on having the right technology in place—but not just for "data capture" or "analysis." **The real power of technology is how it makes your marketing *work in the real world*.**

When your systems make it easy to track where leads come from, follow up quickly, and keep patients engaged, your marketing becomes a predictable process that brings in the *right* patients—the ones who align with your philosophy and stay committed to treatment.

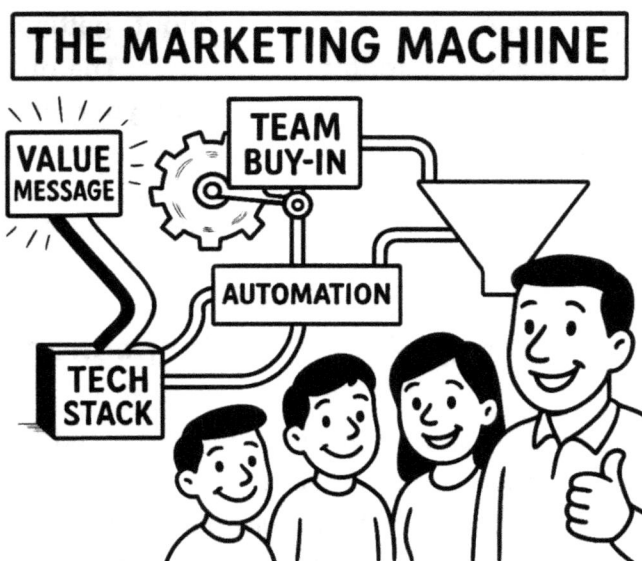

THE MARKETING MACHINE

VALUE MESSAGE

TEAM BUY-IN

AUTOMATION

TECH STACK

Technology bridges the gap between your message and the patient's experience. It ensures the promise you make in your ads is the reality they feel when they walk through your door. It allows you to follow up with those who weren't ready today and convert them when they are. It helps you see which campaigns are working and where to double down.

Every investment you make in technology amplifies the impact of your marketing. The two work together, creating not just growth but sustainable growth that actually makes your practice more enjoyable to run.

Marketing and technology aren't separate silos. They're two sides of the same strategy—helping you build the practice you've always envisioned, with patients you're proud to serve and a team that's empowered to deliver.

The Marketing Magnetism Method: Attracting Your Ideal Patients

Effective marketing is more than growth. It is growth driven by purpose.

When you attract the right patients, you reduce the friction that leads to burnout and build a practice that energizes you instead of draining you. The strategies in this chapter give you a smarter, more sustainable way to grow—one that aligns with your values and your vision.

The framework below turns these ideas into actionable steps you can implement immediately. Each step builds on the last, creating a system that improves over time.

Your Marketing Action Plan

Research your target market (1–2 weeks)

Survey your current patients online and in-office. Ask about demographics, how they found you, and what they value most about your care.

Define your ideal patient profile (2–3 days)

Analyze the results and identify clear patterns. Build a detailed persona—age range, priorities, preferences, and pain points. This becomes your North Star for all marketing decisions.

Craft your unique value proposition (3–5 days)

Write one or two sentences that clearly explain why patients should choose you. Test it with trusted patients or colleagues until it feels authentic and resonates.

Develop your multi-channel strategy (1 week)

Pick three or four marketing channels based on where your ideal patients spend their time. Allocate your budget strategically so each channel gets the focus it needs.

Create your content calendar (2–3 days)

Plan three months of content addressing the questions and concerns your ideal patients have. Keep your voice consistent and tied to your unique value proposition.

Track performance metrics (Ongoing, weekly review)

Monitor website analytics, patient inquiries, and conversion rates. Document what messages and channels perform best.

Refine and reallocate (Monthly)

Every month, review the data. Double down on what works, cut what doesn't, and reallocate your resources accordingly. Be ruthless.

Leverage social proof (Ongoing)

Actively collect testimonials and reviews from satisfied patients who fit your ideal profile. Make it easy for them to share their story on your chosen platforms.

The beauty of this system is its self-correcting nature. **By measuring and adjusting consistently, your marketing gets sharper, more efficient, and more effective at attracting the patients you actually want to serve.**

Technology amplifies these efforts. The right tech stack reinforces your value proposition throughout the patient journey— from automated reminders that respect their time to portals that improve communication and transparency. These touchpoints build trust and support your marketing at every step.

And remember: marketing is never truly "finished." The best practices treat it as an ongoing conversation with their community, refining and adjusting based on feedback and results.

When you market with intention—not just for attention— you create a sustainable growth engine that aligns with your vision and values.

By following the steps in this chapter, you're building relationships with the right patients, the ones who appreciate what you do and make practicing more rewarding.

These are the patients who become the foundation of the practice you've always dreamed of.

Key Takeaways

- Marketing is not a magic bullet. It only works when supported by systems, culture, and team alignment.

- Technology amplifies good marketing, but it cannot replace the clarity of a message or a well-defined process.

- The most effective marketing reflects your practice's personality and values, creating alignment between who you are and who you attract.

- Sustainable growth comes from attracting the right patients, not just more patients.

- Treat marketing partners as collaborators, not vendors. Feedback and integration are essential.

Next Steps

You don't have to wait for a big budget or a perfect system to start marketing with intention. Starting this week, you can:

Review your last marketing investment – Ask whether it aligned with your culture, your team's strengths, and your practice personality.

Involve your team – Before adopting any new tool or campaign, explain its purpose, provide proper training, and gather their input on how it will impact their workflow.

Clarify your value proposition – Write down, in one or two sentences, why patients should choose you. Use it to test whether your marketing message is clear and consistent.

Once you've nailed down your marketing, the real key is to ensure you attract the *right* patients–those who align with the vision of your practice and the life you want outside of it. Marketing should create freedom, not trap you in a practice that drains you. When your message brings in patients who energize your team, appreciate your approach, and value the experience you deliver, they become loyal advocates who refer others and fuel sustainable growth. In the next chapter, we'll explore the new patient journey—how to design intake and onboarding systems that turn the right leads into lasting relationships and ensure your marketing efforts support the practice you truly want to build.

Chapter 7: The New Patient Journey

By: Luke Infinger

Dr. John stared at the production report on his desk. Collections were solid. New patient starts were steady. By all the usual measures, the practice was doing well.

So why did it feel like he was drowning?

Every day was the same: an overbooked schedule, constant interruptions, rushed conversations with patients, and late dinners at home, too distracted to enjoy. No matter how hard he worked, there was no sense of progress—just more of the same.

John wasn't sinking. But he wasn't moving forward either. He was treading water.

And that's the danger so many clinicians face. Growth without boundaries will consume you. The real question isn't how many new patients you can attract. It's about defining what "enough" looks like and then designing the new patient journey to support it. When you intentionally build systems that attract, qualify, and convert the right patients, you stop chasing endless growth and start building a sustainable practice that fuels both your success and your freedom.

Your marketing, technology, and messaging bring attention to your practice and attract the kinds of patients you most want to serve. What happens after a patient raises their hand determines whether you create a practice that supports your vision or one that consumes it.

That's where the new patient journey comes in. It's the handoff point where external growth meets internal operations, and where clarity about your boundaries becomes the difference between thriving and burning out.

This chapter unpacks how to design your new patient journey with intention. From the moment an inquiry comes in, to the first phone call, to the consultation itself, every step is an opportunity to align your growth with your goals. We'll explore how to establish boundaries that protect your time and energy, how to systematize intake and consultations for both efficiency and trust, and how to utilize technology to support, not replace, the human connection your patients need most.

When you master this journey, growth stops feeling like a burden and starts fueling the life and practice you've always envisioned.

When "Enough" Stops Being Fuzzy and Starts Being Freedom

For orthodontists and dentists, growth is the gospel we're sold from the start. More patients. More chairs. More revenue. More recognition.

But here's the uncomfortable truth: **almost no one ever stops to ask what "enough" actually looks like**—for *you*.

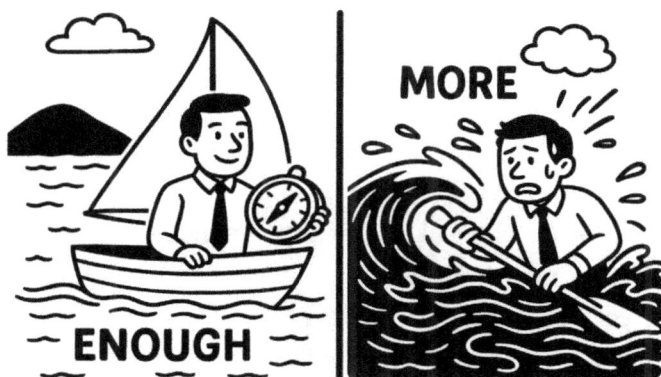

Without clearly defined boundaries and goals, most practices are like ships without a rudder. They drift. They chase whatever current seems strongest. And before long, the practice you built to give you freedom starts to feel like the thing that owns you.

This chapter is about fixing that.

We're going to zero in on one of the most overlooked—and most important—systems in your practice: the new patient journey. This is where marketing hands off to operations, and where your future growth either aligns with your vision or derails it completely.

The goal isn't just to "convert more leads." That's short-sighted. The goal is to design a process that intentionally attracts, qualifies, and converts *the right patients*—and to do it in a way that matches the outcomes you've set for your life and your practice.

As Brian Tracy says, *"Goals are the fuel in the furnace of achievement."* **But goals without boundaries are dangerous. Every clinician we talk to wants "more," yet 99.5% of them have no clear idea of what they're chasing or why.**

Success leaves clues. Look at the practices in your market and identify one that reflects the lifestyle, schedule, and culture you truly want, not just the one posting the biggest numbers. Study what they prioritize and, just as importantly, what they intentionally avoid.

From there, define your own goals and boundaries. Put them in writing. Be crystal clear about the outcome you're chasing and the reason behind it. Then design your intake and patient acquisition systems to align with that vision instead of blindly pursuing growth for growth's sake.

Define 'enough' not just emotionally but numerically. Clarify how many new patient starts you need each month, the conversion rate you aim for, and how many consultations that requires. For example, if you want 50 starts a month at a 75% conversion rate, you'll need about 67 consultations scheduled. This helps you measure progress and set clear, realistic boundaries.

Because the systems that help you grow your patient base can either liberate you or consume you. And you get to decide which.

The Boundary Paradox

Counterintuitively, establishing boundaries around your practice focuses growth rather than restricting it.

When you define what "enough" means for your schedule, your revenue, and your lifestyle, you gain clarity about which patients deserve your attention and which systems deserve your investment. The most successful orthodontists and dentists we've worked with don't chase every possible lead. They've built intentional intake processes that align with their vision of a balanced, sustainable practice. This reflects an abundance mindset, one that focuses not on scarcity and competition but on attracting and converting the right patients while maintaining healthy growth and balance. Defining enough helps you step into this mindset with clarity and confidence.

In the pages ahead, we'll unpack three foundational elements of an effective new patient journey. First, how to implement a fast-response and pre-qualification system to convert inquiries into consults quickly while maintaining alignment with your goals. Second, how to structure a streamlined new patient exam with a focus on influence-driven scripting and same-day start opportunities. Third, which technologies and tracking systems such as a CRM and virtual consultations streamline the process without depersonalizing it.

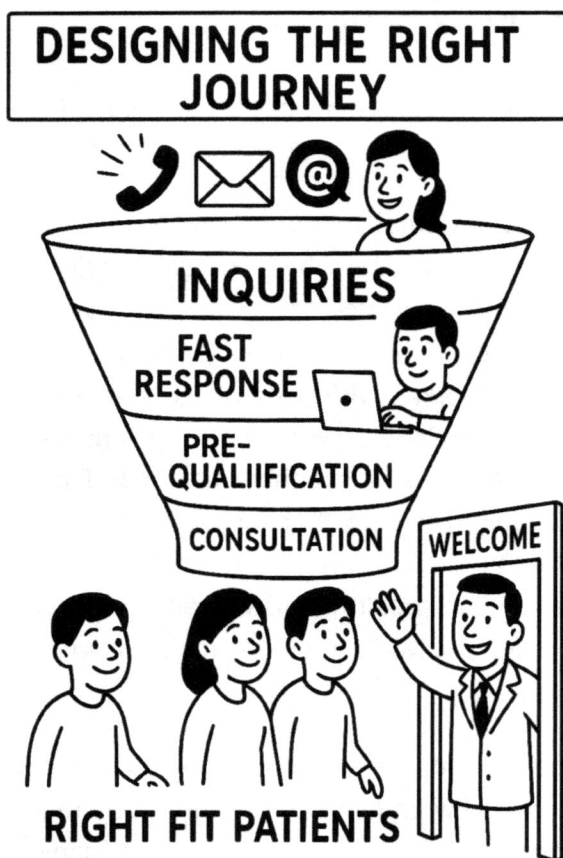

DESIGNING THE RIGHT JOURNEY

INQUIRIES

FAST RESPONSE

PRE-QUALIIFICATION

CONSULTATION

WELCOME

RIGHT FIT PATIENTS

For example, a CRM like PracticeBeacon can help you track pending patients and follow-ups systematically, while virtual consultations can save chair time and help qualify patients before they walk in.

This isn't just about efficiency—though you'll gain that too. It's about taking back control of your growth trajectory. When you clearly define what "enough" means to you—in patients, in revenue, in fulfillment—you create space for your own well-being.

The most sustainable practices are the ones designed thoughtfully to support your ambitions and your life outside the office.

The systems we'll explore are more like boundaries in disguise than your typical set of administrative tools. Each one helps protect you from the kind of unchecked expansion that turns a dream practice into a daily grind.

These systems work best when each team member understands and owns their role in the journey. Front desk staff should respond to leads quickly and pre-qualify patients to reduce no-shows. Treatment Coordinators should follow a clear consultation script and fee presentation that builds confidence and makes same-day starts feel natural. The clinical team should be prepared to seat same-day starts efficiently. When everyone contributes to the process, the entire practice stays aligned with your defined boundaries.

Mastering the new patient journey, within the context of your own "enough," lays the foundation for a practice that enhances your life instead of consuming it.

Remember: the goal isn't to build the biggest practice possible. It's to build the practice that best serves your definition of a meaningful life.

Let's dive in.

The Day Dr. John Stopped Treading Water

Dr. John thought back to his first year out of residency, when every milestone felt exciting—the first 100 patients, the first million in production, the first associate he hired. But now? The numbers kept climbing, yet the joy had drained away.

It wasn't that his practice was failing—it was that he had never defined what success should actually look like. More patients. More revenue. More growth. But to what end? Each new "win" only seemed to add more weight to his shoulders.

Late one evening, after another long day and another missed dinner at home, John pulled out a notebook. He drew two columns: Enough and Excess. Under Enough, he wrote down clear, measurable boundaries—how many patients he wanted to start each month, how many hours he wanted to work, and what kind of schedule would let him be present for his family. Under Excess, he listed the things he was no longer willing to tolerate: double-booked days, late-night charting, and saying yes to patients who didn't fit the practice he envisioned.

> That exercise was the turning point. For the first time in years, John wasn't just surviving his practice—he was reshaping it.

Moral: Without clear goals and boundaries, even a "successful" practice can leave you feeling stuck. The day you define what *enough* looks like is the day you start moving forward on your own terms.

Inquiry to Appointment: Building Systems That Convert

Every practice gets inquiries—by phone, email, website forms, and now social media. But thriving practices don't just attract leads. They convert them.

Your intake process is the front door to your practice. When a potential patient knocks, does it open smoothly and make them feel welcome? Or does it stick, creak, and frustrate them? First impressions start long before they step inside.

High conversion takes both systems and a human touch. The best practices use standardized protocols that ensure fast, consistent responses while keeping interactions personal. These often include scripts for common questions, follow-up templates, and clear tracking from first contact to booked appointment.

Speed matters. Research shows responding to a lead within five minutes makes them 100 times more likely to convert than if you wait just 30 minutes. In our field, where patients reach out during moments of stress or worry, quick reassurance is everything.

Every unnecessary step or delay creates friction—and friction sends people elsewhere. Audit your intake process regularly and ask: *Does this step help the patient, or just make our admin feel better?* Eliminate what you can.

One practice I worked with increased their scheduled appointments by 20% in just two months by making one simple change. Instead of asking patients when they wanted to come in, their team began offering appointments within 72 hours during the very first call. That sense of urgency and clarity turned more conversations into commitments.

Language also matters. Tone and tempo are everything on a phone call. In fact, only about 7% of communication is the actual words you say. The way you say it—your tone, pace, and energy—is what establishes rapport and trust.

Your team should use empathetic, patient-centered phrasing that builds certainty and reassurance. Lines like *"I totally understand how that feels"* and *"So that you don't have to worry about…"* make patients feel heard, valued, and confident they've called the right practice.

Track your results. Monitor inquiry-to-appointment ratio, average response time, and conversion rate by lead source. Those numbers reveal exactly where your process shines and where it needs work.

And don't forget: not every lead is ready today. Most practices leave money on the table by ignoring those "not yet" prospects. A simple nurturing sequence—check-in calls, helpful emails—keeps you top-of-mind for when they're ready to move forward.

Your intake system should act as both a filter and a funnel. It brings the right patients in quickly while setting the tone for a relationship built on trust and care.

First Impressions: The Foundation of Patient Relationships

The first interaction with a new patient should set expectations, build trust, and lay the foundation for the entire relationship. Get it right, and you increase retention, satisfaction, and even clinical outcomes.

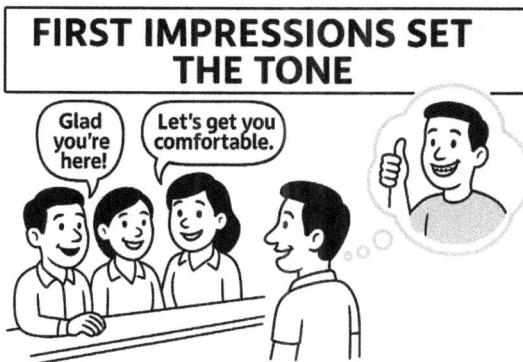

Patient psychology is clear: the impressions formed during that first interaction heavily shape how patients perceive all future care—and those perceptions are remarkably hard to change. A patient who feels rushed, confused, or unheard during their first contact will carry that feeling into every visit, even if your clinical work is flawless.

Why does this happen? Because people entering a new environment are vulnerable and uncertain. They're looking for clues about what kind of experience they're about to have—and those early signals become anchors in their mind for everything that follows.

Think of these first interactions like the foundation of a building. You can build something beautiful on top, but if the foundation is cracked, the whole structure is compromised over time.

Exceptional first impressions meet both practical and emotional needs. Patients need clarity about logistics, costs, and what to expect. But just as important, they need reassurance, empathy, and confidence that you can help. Neglect either, and the relationship starts on shaky ground.

One small orthodontic practice I worked with cut no-shows by 17% and boosted satisfaction scores simply by adding a five-minute "connection call" 1–2 days before a patient's first appointment. The team confirmed logistics, answered simple questions, and—most importantly—put a warm, human voice to the practice before the patient even walked in.

When the patient does arrive, your physical space and process either reinforce or undermine the impression you've made. Is your reception area clean and aligned with the image you project online? Does check-in feel seamless and expected? When what patients see matches what they've been told, trust deepens. When it doesn't, doubt creeps in.

The stakes are real. Research from the Cleveland Clinic found that patients with positive first impressions were 36% more likely to follow through on their treatment plan and reported 28% higher satisfaction—even when the actual clinical care was identical.

Technology can enhance, but not replace, this critical moment. Digital intake forms, automated text reminders with parking details, and welcome videos from the doctor can all reduce anxiety and build familiarity. But no app can substitute for a caring tone, a smile at the front desk, and staff who make the patient feel seen.

If you stopped treating first interactions like a box to check and started treating them as the most important part of the patient journey, how different might your relationships and results look?

Technology as the Enabler of Administrative Excellence

Administrative tasks eat up an enormous share of time and energy in a dental or orthodontic practice. **Studies show clinicians spend 20–40% of their workweek on paperwork rather than patient care.** That burden fuels burnout, drags down revenue, and kills job satisfaction.

But done right, technology changes that.

Patient intake is one of the easiest wins. Digital forms eliminate redundant data entry, cut down on errors, and let patients fill everything out at home instead of clogging your waiting room. Better systems even sync directly with your practice management software, so staff don't have to retype a thing.

Here's the catch: too many practices just digitize their clunky old process instead of rethinking it. That's not progress. The right way to approach it is to start with your desired outcome, design a smarter workflow, and then use technology to support it.

Take scheduling. Phone-based scheduling wastes staff time, creates bottlenecks during busy hours, and frustrates patients who can't get through. A good online scheduling platform lets patients see openings and book anytime—no calls required. Pair it with automated reminders and you'll cut no-shows and lighten the load on your team.

Think of technology like a transit system. Even the nicest highway is useless if it doesn't take people where they need to go, or if the on-ramps are impossible to navigate. The best software is only as good as how it's implemented—it needs to solve your specific problems and be easy enough for staff and patients to actually use.

Communication is another area where technology shines. Secure messaging platforms I.e, Rhinogram, cut down on endless phone calls and keep a record of patient conversations. Automated reminders and mass messaging tools make it easy to announce closures, policy changes, or upcoming events without eating up staff time.

On the financial side, digital payment options improve cash flow while reducing headaches. Patient portals, card-on-file setups, and automated billing reminders take the burden off staff—and many practices report a 15–30% increase in collections after switching.

Document management tools also save time and space. Cloud-based systems securely store and organize forms, images, and records so staff can retrieve and share them instantly—no more digging through file cabinets or wasting time on photocopies.

Here's the hard truth: the biggest barrier to effective technology isn't the software. It's the people. Staff get comfortable with old habits. If they don't understand why the change matters or they don't feel trained and supported, they'll resist.

That's why successful practices don't just drop new tools on the team. They take time to explain how it ties into the bigger goals of the practice—more time for patients, less busywork, less stress—and provide solid training and ongoing support.

The point isn't to replace human connection with automation. It's to clear the clutter so your team can focus where it counts—building relationships, delivering care, and growing the kind of practice you actually want to run.

Bringing It All Together: The Patient Engagement Ecosystem

Lead intake. First impressions. Administrative technology.

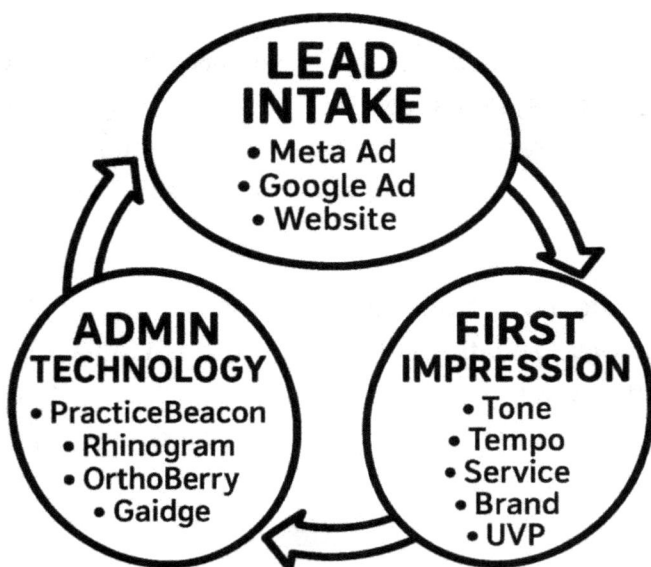

LEAD INTAKE
- Meta Ad
- Google Ad
- Website

FIRST IMPRESSION
- Tone
- Tempo
- Service
- Brand
- UVP

ADMIN TECHNOLOGY
- PracticeBeacon
- Rhinogram
- OrthoBerry
- Gaidge

This interconnected system makes up one key tool: your patient engagement ecosystem.

When these elements work in harmony, they create a seamless experience that attracts the right patients, converts them efficiently, and builds lasting relationships. Just as important, they let you define what enough looks like for your practice—and stick to it. That's how you grow without burning out.

The best practices understand that every patient touchpoint, from first click to final follow-up, needs to reflect who you are and what you stand for. Every interaction—your website, your phone calls, your waiting room, your team's language—should send the same message: here's what we're about, and here's how we can help.

That kind of consistency builds trust and keeps patients from experiencing the disconnect that happens when what they see online doesn't match what they feel in your office.

As you build your ecosystem, think in terms of appropriate automation. Automate the routine. Personalize the meaningful. Technology is great for things like reminders, forms, and scheduling—but it can never replace the human connection patients feel when your team greets them warmly and listens attentively.

And always come back to this: **your systems aren't just there to fill your chairs. They're there to bring in the right patients—the ones who value your care, fit your philosophy, and make your practice more fulfilling to run.**

When designed with intention, your patient engagement ecosystem becomes the blueprint for a sustainable, thriving practice. One that grows on your terms, serves your patients well, and respects your boundaries.

That's the power of doing this work on purpose—not just more, but better.

Finding Your Conversion Sweet Spot

Every practice sits somewhere on the spectrum of lead conversion effectiveness. At one extreme are practices so obsessed with efficiency they come off cold and rigid—patients feel like they're being processed, not welcomed. At the other are warm, friendly practices with such chaotic systems they drop leads, miss follow-ups, and frustrate patients with friction.

The sweet spot sits right in the middle: reliable systems paired with authentic human connection.

That balance allows you to consistently deliver excellent first impressions without demanding heroics from your team. It lets you scale while preserving the quality that makes your practice stand out.

Start by honestly assessing where you are today. Ask yourself:

- Do inquiries get prompt, helpful responses?

- Is scheduling straightforward or inefficient?

- Are leads falling through the cracks?

- Do new patients arrive feeling informed, valued, and confident they made the right choice?

Many clinicians avoid systematizing their intake because they worry it will feel "corporate" or impersonal. That's a misunderstanding.

Well-built systems do not prevent connection. They create the structure that allows connection to thrive.

When your team isn't scrambling to remember what comes next or searching for information, they have the bandwidth to focus on what matters: the person in front of them.

Here's a simple framework to evaluate your conversion process:

1. **Responsiveness** – How fast do you acknowledge an inquiry?

2. **Clarity** – Can patients easily understand your services, next steps, and expectations?

3. **Convenience** – How simple is it to schedule, complete forms, or get questions answered?

4. **Connection** – Do patients feel personally seen and understood?

5. **Consistency** – Does every patient get the same excellent experience?

Improving any of these areas will raise your conversion rates—usually fast. More importantly, these improvements ripple throughout the entire patient journey, because first impressions set the tone for everything that follows.

And remember: conversion isn't about manipulating people into saying yes. It's about making it easy for the right patients to move forward—and making sure the fit is mutual.

The Psychology of New Patient Consults

First appointments carry more weight than most clinicians realize.

For patients, they're a mix of hope, vulnerability, and evaluation. They're asking themselves: Can I trust you? Do you understand me? Do I feel comfortable here?

For you, it's a balancing act: assess clinically, build a relationship, and set expectations—all in one encounter.

And these moments matter. Research from the *Journal of Medical Practice Management* shows that 96% of patient complaints come from service failures, not clinical care. The top issues? Feeling rushed, not being heard, and unclear next steps. All common mistakes during first appointments.

Patients arrive carrying invisible concerns. Many have had bad experiences with other providers. Others worry about being judged, fear the cost, or dread what you might find. Acknowledging those concerns—even before they're spoken—immediately sets you apart.

How you structure the consult matters. Too often, doctors dive straight into the clinical and skip establishing rapport and vision. A better approach looks like this:

- Start with connection and future pacing: *"I've reviewed your intake and see you're dealing with [x]. Can you tell me more about how this has been affecting you— and what you're hoping to achieve by the end of treatment?"*

   This not only validates their current experience but also gets them to articulate their desired outcome, creating buy-in and shared focus.

- Move into your clinical evaluation: explain findings and options in the context of the outcome they described.

- End by clearly outlining next steps and reinforcing their vision: tie the plan back to their goal—"This is the first step toward getting you to [desired result]."

By framing the conversation around where the patient wants to end up, you help them see your treatment as a pathway to their personal goal, not just a set of procedures. That simple shift increases trust, motivation, and compliance.

Whenever possible, offer patients the opportunity to start treatment the same day as their consultation. This reduces decision fatigue, aligns with the momentum they already feel walking in, and keeps conversion rates high—a proven strategy used by top-performing practices.

Your environment matters too. Does your office feel welcoming or cold? Are there private areas for sensitive conversations? Even small details—noise, temperature, seating—shape how patients perceive your competence and care.

One practice improved their treatment acceptance rates simply by adding five minutes at the end of each first appointment to ask: "What questions haven't I answered yet?" and "What concerns do you have about the plan we discussed?" That small step made a big difference.

The initial consult also sets the tone for how patients interact with your practice. Be clear about communication, scheduling, payments, and what you expect from them going forward. This prevents future friction and builds confidence.

And remember: how patients leave matters as much as how they arrive. A rushed ending with unanswered questions can undo an otherwise excellent appointment. A clear, confident close builds trust and momentum.

Even if a patient doesn't move forward right away, their experience still matters. Those who feel respected often refer others or come back later when the timing is right. Those who feel dismissed rarely do.

Every new patient exam is an opportunity to earn trust today—
and to build your reputation for tomorrow.

Technology That Serves Rather Than Dominates

Technology fails when we forget its purpose: to serve human needs, not dictate human behavior.

In healthcare, the point of technology is to enhance the human connection that defines great care. Every administrative tech decision you make should be grounded in that principle.

The most effective implementations start with the right question: *What problem are we solving?* Too many practices get dazzled by impressive demos or trade show pitches, only to end up with expensive tools that don't actually address their real needs.

Most practices see the greatest gains from technologies that improve these core areas:

- Patient communication: secure messaging, automated reminders, mass notifications.

- Documentation: digital forms, e-signatures, organized document storage.

- Scheduling: online booking, real-time availability, efficient resource allocation.

- Payments: online portals, automated billing, clear policy management.

- Patient experience: streamlined check-in, satisfaction surveys, review requests.

Always weigh how well a system integrates. Standalone tools that can't talk to each other often create more work than they eliminate. Even the flashiest app is worthless if it forces duplicate entry or manual reconciliation.

Also account for the true cost of implementation—not just subscription fees, but training time, workflow disruption, and the bandwidth required to support it. Fancy software that never gets fully adopted can bleed a practice dry.

Involving your staff early on is critical. They'll spot real-world challenges decision-makers often miss. Plus, their buy-in creates internal advocates who help others through the transition. In contrast, tools imposed top-down without staff input almost always meet quiet resistance.

Balance is key: too rigid a system frustrates everyone when exceptions arise. Too flexible a system breeds inconsistency. The best solutions hit the sweet spot—structured enough to be reliable, flexible enough to work in reality.

One mid-sized practice we partnered with learned this the hard way. They spent over $30,000 and countless staff hours implementing a new practice management software—only to abandon it. Why? It was overbuilt for their needs and too complex to use. What had impressed them in the demo turned out to work properly and overall, the software wasn't best for their workflow.

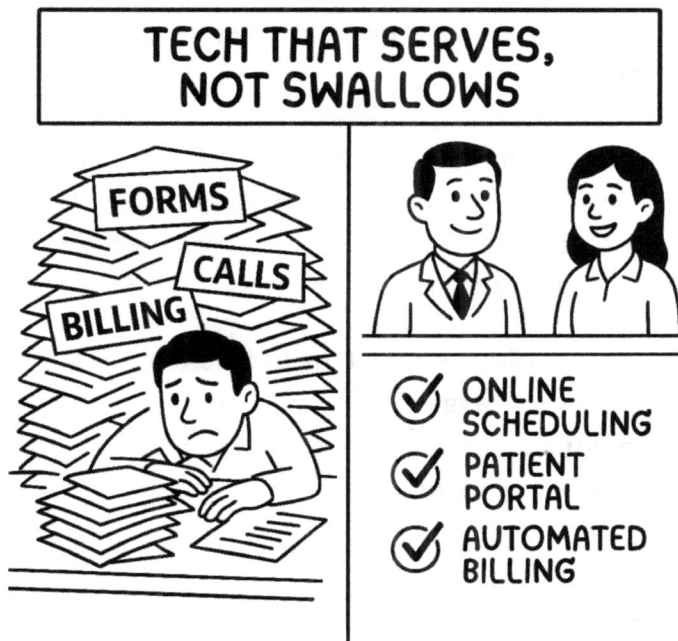

TECH THAT SERVES, NOT SWALLOWS

FORMS
CALLS
BILLING

✓ ONLINE SCHEDULING
✓ PATIENT PORTAL
✓ AUTOMATED BILLING

When evaluating technology, ask:

- How intuitive is it—for both staff and patients?

- What training and support does the vendor offer?

- How have they handled security issues in the past?

- What's the realistic implementation timeline?

- How easy is it to export your data if you ever switch?

- Can it adapt to your workflows without endless customization?

- How responsive is their customer service when things break?

A phased rollout beats a big-bang launch every time. Introducing new tools one step at a time lets your team gain confidence, reveals unexpected challenges early, and avoids overwhelming your operation.

The best technologies aren't the flashiest or most feature-packed. They solve real problems, stay in the background, and free your team to focus where it matters most—on the people sitting in your chairs.

Integration: The Multiplier Effect

Optimizing lead conversion, first impressions, and administrative technology individually creates value. But when you weave them together into a single, integrated system, the impact multiplies. Integration doesn't just improve efficiency—it elevates the entire patient experience.

Here's how it looks in practice:

A patient submits an online inquiry form. They instantly receive a confirmation email and text with helpful educational resources, and your intake coordinator is alerted. The scheduler calls within 5 minutes, using tailored prompts based on what the patient wrote in their form. Once scheduled, the patient gets digital intake paperwork that feeds directly into your health record, eliminating redundant data entry. Automated reminders reduce no-shows. When the patient arrives, your team already knows their history and concerns, and greets them personally. (This could happen with a number of tools working together, i.e., PracticeBeacon, Rhinogram, and OrthoBerry, to name a few.)

That kind of seamless journey builds trust and confidence before the first clinical interaction.

Now contrast that with a fragmented system. Lead management, intake, and admin tools operate in silos. Information gets lost. Staff scramble to double-check or manually re-enter data. Patients repeat themselves to multiple people. That friction undermines confidence, wastes time, and drives up costs.

Integration doesn't mean you have to buy one expensive, all-in-one platform. Many practices successfully connect best-in-class tools using middleware or integration services. The key is designing workflows where information flows cleanly from one step to the next, minimizing manual handoffs. Even partial integration is a massive improvement over disconnected systems.

Pay special attention to the handoff between admin and clinical teams. Patients routinely complain: "Why am I telling the doctor the same thing I already told the front desk?" Tight integration ensures information flows seamlessly—while still giving clinicians the chance to verify what they need.

When done well, integration becomes a force multiplier. It removes friction, builds trust, and frees your team to deliver their best work.

Defining "Enough" in Your Administrative Systems

Everything we've covered in this chapter—better systems, smarter technology, seamless integration—is only valuable if it serves your definition of enough.

Administrative excellence is about creating a practice that works efficiently at the *right* patient volume, not endlessly chasing more.

What "enough" looks like will vary.

- A solo doctor may value simplicity and systems that save their time.

- A growing practice may focus on scalability and structure.

- A mature practice may emphasize consistency and refinement.

Systems that fit your vision rather than arbitrary sales pitches or even industry benchmarks are always a step ahead.

Ask yourself:

- Do our systems support the patient volume we actually want?

- Do they create room for the meaningful work that drew me into this field?

- Do they free my mind for growth, learning, and life outside the office?

If the answer is yes, then you've already hit "enough"—even if your metrics aren't maximized.

Administrative technology, in particular, demands discernment. Every month brings a new "must-have" tool. But every addition increases complexity. Sometimes the best move is to keep things simple—even at the cost of a little efficiency—if it means your systems remain manageable and aligned with your goals.

When you evaluate a potential improvement, don't just ask *Will this make things better?*

Ask: *Will this make things better in a way that matters to me and my practice?*

That simple question keeps you out of the trap of optimizing for its own sake—a trap that can leave you with a "perfect" system that doesn't serve your life.

The best administrative systems are the ones that let you run the practice you actually want, at the pace you actually want, with the freedom and boundaries you actually need.

That's the real definition of enough.

Mastering the First Impression: Beyond Admin to Patient Connection

New patient intake is the foundation of your practice's sustainability and your personal well-being.

Throughout this chapter, we've shown how your systems directly shape your ability to define and maintain your "enough."

When you build reliable conversion systems, optimize those critical first interactions, and implement the right technology, you're doing more than streamlining operations. You're creating space to practice on your own terms.

The truth is simple and liberating: without clear boundaries around what "enough" looks like—in patients, revenue, or satisfaction—the default becomes more. And "more" is the fastest route to burnout.

Every new patient relationship starts long before they walk into your office. The systems you design now determine whether you spend your days drowning in chaos or fully present with the people who need you most.

This is really about freedom.

Freedom to focus on quality over quantity.

Freedom to build meaningful connections rather than rush through checklists.

Freedom to leave on time, knowing your systems keep running without you.

The clinicians who thrive over decades are the ones who defined "enough," and built systems to honor it.

As you refine your lead intake and administrative processes, keep asking:

Does this support my vision of having enough? Or is it just pushing me toward more?

That answer will tell you if you're building the practice you dreamed of—or just finding a more efficient path to burnout.

The systems you implement today will define the practice, and the life you live tomorrow.

Make them intentional.

Make them efficient.

And most of all—make them yours.

Key Takeaways

- Growth without boundaries leads to exhaustion. Defining "enough" creates clarity and freedom.
- The new patient journey is more than conversion. It's about filtering for fit and aligning with your long-term goals.
- Systems work best when every team member owns their role, ensuring fast responses, empathetic communication, structured consults, and same-day starts.
- Technology is a multiplier only when implemented thoughtfully and integrated seamlessly with your workflows.
- Success isn't the biggest practice. It's the one aligned with your vision of a meaningful life.

Next Steps

You don't have to rebuild your patient journey overnight. Starting this week, you can:

Define your "enough" – Write down your target starts, conversion rate, and the schedule you want to sustain.

Audit your intake process – Track response times, conversion rates, and friction points from first inquiry to consult.

Improve one first impression touchpoint – Add a connection call, redesign your consult script, or streamline scheduling.

Involve your team – Clarify roles in the journey so every step, from first call to treatment start, has an owner.

Once you've defined the patient journey that reflects both your ideal practice and the life you want to live, the next step is making sure patients actually move through that journey with confidence. It's not enough to attract the right leads—you have to help them say "yes" in a way that supports your boundaries and your profitability.

That's where treatment coordination and sales come in. Mastering this part of the process ensures you're not just filling chairs but converting the *right number* of the *right patients* into starts. Done well, treatment coordination maximizes the true value of every lead, strengthens trust, and creates the financial foundation that allows your practice to thrive without consuming you.

In the next chapter, we'll look at how to reframe sales as service, how to calculate the real lifetime value of each patient, and how to build systems that capture the full worth of every opportunity that walks through your door.

Chapter 8: Treatment Coordination and Sales

By: Dr. Kyle Fagala

Dr. Jennifer's practice looked like a success story. Her case acceptance rate was an enviable 92%, the highest in her study club. Colleagues asked for her secrets. Consultants used her as an example. But behind the numbers, something didn't add up.

Despite seeing more patients than ever, her take-home income had dropped. The "patient-friendly" policies she'd adopted—accepting every insurance, eliminating down payments, and stretching payment terms—had boosted her conversion rate but gutted her profitability. She was working harder than ever, yet her financial stress was rising.

Jennifer had fallen into the conversion rate trap.

This chapter reveals the paradox at the heart of treatment coordination: what looks like success on paper often traps you in a cycle of more work for less reward. Conversion rate alone is a misleading metric. The true measure is the lifetime value of each patient and the profitability of each start. When you and your team master treatment coordination and sales ethically, you stop chasing vanity numbers and start building a practice that is both financially sustainable and deeply fulfilling.

In this chapter, we'll uncover how to calculate the true value of each patient, avoid the conversion rate trap, and implement systems from the doctorless consult to the Perfect Consult™ framework that make treatment acceptance both natural and ethical. Done right, treatment coordination doesn't just increase starts, it builds a stronger practice that supports the life you want to live.

The $4,700 Question That Changes Everything

Picture this: You're walking to your car after a long day, and there's a bundle of $100 bills worth $4,700 just sitting on the asphalt. Would you bend down to pick it up?

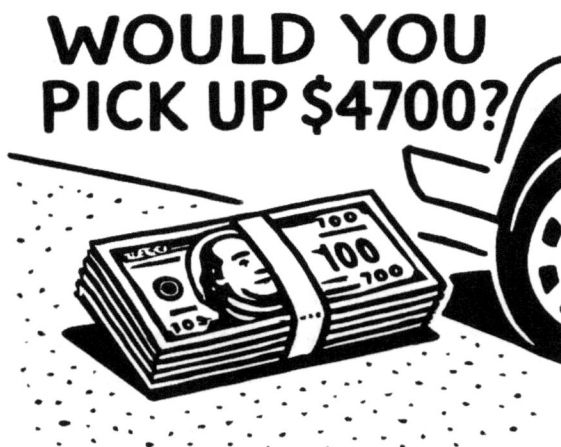

WOULD YOU PICK UP $4700?

Of course you would.

Yet every day, orthodontists and their team members let that exact amount go unscheduled or even walk out their front door because they don't understand a fundamental truth: **that's what every qualified lead is worth to your practice.**

Most clinicians obsess over conversion rates—the percentage of consultations that turn into treatment. But here's the reality check that changes everything: **conversion rate is actually a limiting metric that can lead you to make terrible business decisions.**

What matters isn't how many people say "yes." What matters is how much money you take home after the right people say "yes."

Dr. Jennifer didn't realize the truth of her situation until we guided her to calculate the lifetime value of each patient.

On paper, her acceptance rate looked incredible. But when she ran the numbers, the picture changed. Her profit per case had dropped 31% since adopting all those "patient-friendly" policies. In her effort to make treatment accessible to everyone—accepting every insurance, eliminating down payments, and stretching payment terms—

she had built a machine that looked successful but left her exhausted and financially strained.

High acceptance wasn't the problem. It was what she'd sacrificed to get it.

By treating every consultation as if it were worth $47 instead of the $4,700 it truly represented, Jennifer had filled her schedule with patients who drained her resources and left little margin for the growth and freedom she'd once envisioned.

The clincher? Her practice wasn't failing because she wasn't converting enough leads. It was failing because she hadn't defined which patients she actually wanted to say 'yes', and at what value.

Why Every Great Dentist Must Master the Art of the Close

The moment your patient leans back in that chair, it's already happening. The relationship building. The trust formation. The groundwork for acceptance of your clinical recommendations.

In dental school, they taught you to diagnose conditions and perform procedures with precision—but they likely skipped the chapter on how to help patients commit to the treatment they genuinely need while building a sustainable and profitable practice.

Treatment coordination is where clinical excellence meets practice sustainability. When done properly, it transforms the experience for everyone involved. Your patients receive the comprehensive care they need. Your team feels the satisfaction of serving completely. Your practice generates the revenue necessary to invest in better equipment, continuing education, and the compensation everyone deserves.

The discomfort many clinicians feel around the financial aspects of treatment speaks to a deeper paradox. We enter healthcare professions with noble intentions to heal and help, only to discover that our ability to deliver that care depends on business acumen that wasn't part of our training.

The Lifetime Value Revolution

Most practices dramatically undervalue their patients because they only calculate initial case fees. But smart business owners think differently.

Here's the real math that changes how you approach every consultation:

For orthodontists with an average case fee of $6,180 and a conservatively high overhead of 60%, each treatment start generates approximately $2,472 in profit. But that's just the beginning.

The lifetime value actually includes:

- Initial treatment profit: $2,472
- Retreatment (1 in ~40 patients): Additional $2,000+ profit
- Replacement retainers and accessories: $500 average over the patient's lifetime
- Referrals from satisfied patients: 2-3 additional starts
- **Total lifetime value: $6,500-$12,000 per patient**

Chris Bentson, a well-respected expert in the orthodontic field, suggests a lifetime value near 2x the case fee (~$10,000+), though conservatively, $6,500–$12,000 is a realistic estimate.

When you multiply this by your 70% average conversion rate, **every qualified lead walking through your door is worth** (from a conservative point of view) approximately $4,700.

Now the question becomes: Are you treating $4,700 leads like they're worth $47 or $4,700?

The Conversion Rate Trap That's Killing Your Profitability

Here's the uncomfortable truth that most practice management consultants won't tell you: **conversion rate is a very limiting metric.**

What matters most when it comes to treatment coordination? Take-home dollars and cents.

Charge more for a case, and your conversion rate will go down. But based on research like the **Kodak study**—a landmark business analysis that examined the relationship between pricing strategies and profitability across multiple industries—**you have to do far less work when your case fee and effective profit per case are higher.**

The Kodak study revealed that companies focusing on premium pricing and higher margins consistently outperformed those competing on volume and low prices. In orthodontics, this translates to a crucial insight: it's better to complete 80 high-value cases than 120 low-value cases that exhaust your team and compromise your work-life balance.

Let's be brutally honest about some "successful" strategies:

What's in-network insurance participation? It's just marketing spend where you accept a significantly lower case fee. Surprised your case acceptance is higher when you accept every in-network insurance plan? Of course it is— you're essentially buying patients by giving massive discounts.

Accept $0 down and see your case acceptance rate skyrocket. But what about your collection rate? Your default rate will also skyrocket over time. And your take-home? It will be reduced due to the inefficient and shortsighted approach you decided to take.

Cash flow will also be damaged by myopic decisions that favor getting people to say "yes" instead of focusing on getting the right people to say yes—those who are committed to treatment, to paying on time, and to finishing their payments.

The Doctorless Consultation Revolution

Here's another thing most practices get wrong: they think effective treatment coordination always requires the doctor to be present.

Studies show that practices with dedicated treatment coordinators see case acceptance rates increase by 15-30% on average. This dramatic improvement stems from the coordinator's ability to dedicate uninterrupted time to patient education and address concerns without the clinical pressures faced by doctors.

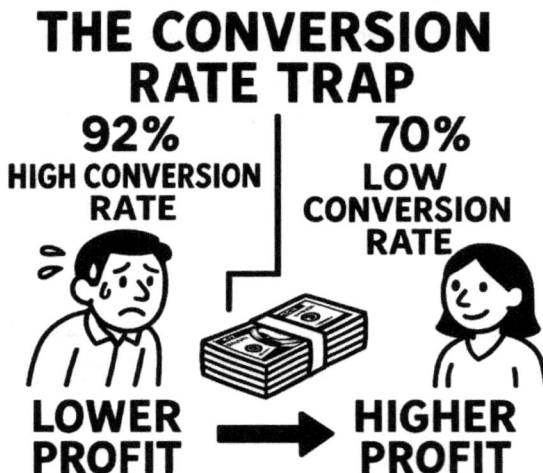

**THE CONVERSION
RATE TRAP**

92%
**HIGH CONVERSION
RATE**

70%
**LOW
CONVERSION
RATE**

**LOWER
PROFIT**   **HIGHER
PROFIT**

The breakthrough insight: properly executed doctorless consultations often outperform traditional models.

Consider your last car-buying experience. What happened when the salesperson left you alone in that room for 20 minutes? You got bored. You started second-guessing. You pulled out your phone to research other options. By the time they returned, your enthusiasm had deflated.

Time kills all deals. And dead time sucks the oxygen out of the sales room.

Imagine a doctor who's always running behind schedule. His treatment coordinator, Lisa, had been trained to follow protocol: always wait for the doctor before presenting financial options. No exceptions.

But when the doctor got stuck in an emergency appointment, Lisa made a bold decision—she presented the financial arrangement herself.

The result? The patient started treatment that day.

When the doctor realized what happened, it became clear that his delays had been creating an unnecessary gap in the patient journey. That pause between consultation and financial discussion was giving patients just enough time to second-guess themselves, to overthink, to lose momentum.

When Lisa maintained the flow from consultation through financial presentation, something shifted. More patients were saying yes. More were starting treatment the same day. The practice began to see what happened when enthusiasm didn't have time to cool.

The lesson? Sometimes the biggest barrier to patient acceptance isn't cost or complexity—it's time. Every moment of delay creates space for doubt to creep in.

Important note: The doctor should always perform an in-person clinical examination before initiating any treatment. However, this clinical exam doesn't have to occur before treatment fees are presented or discussed. A skilled treatment coordinator can present treatment options and financial arrangements based on preliminary assessments, with the understanding that the doctor will confirm the treatment plan during the clinical examination.

The 10 Ps of The Perfect Consult™

After 15 years of practicing orthodontics and countless consultations, I had to face an uncomfortable truth: despite providing excellent clinical care and running a well-designed practice, too many qualified patients were walking out without starting treatment. That's when I developed what I call "The Perfect Consult System"—a 10-step framework that addresses every critical moment of the patient consultation experience.

The problem was the consultation process itself.

THE PERFECT CONSULT SYSTEM

1. THE PEOPLE
2. THE PREPARATION
3. THE PLEASANTRIES
4. THE PROGRAM
5. THE PROBLEM
6. THE PEEK
7. THE PLAN
8. THE PAUSE
9. THE PASS OFF
10. THE PRAYER

P #1: THE PEOPLE

"If the right people aren't on your bus, you cannot have great team culture. If you don't have a great team culture, you'll never be as successful at consults as you could be." – Dr. Kyle

The Hidden Truth: Your team's approach to patient interaction significantly impacts treatment acceptance.

The Perfect People Protocol:

- Hire team members who naturally connect with people
- Make sure everyone understands their role in the patient experience
- Develop consistent approaches to common patient interactions
- Practice handling questions and concerns as a team
- Create systems for continuous improvement

P #2: THE PREPARATION

"Be prepared before new patients ever arrive at your office." – Dr. Kyle

The 5-Minute Pre-Consult Review: Before entering any consultation, briefly consider:

1. What brought them in? (chief complaint)
2. Who will be involved in the decision?
3. Any time-sensitive factors?

4. Previous orthodontic experiences?

5. Any concerns mentioned during scheduling?

P #3: THE PLEASANTRIES

"Be sure to make a great first impression at each step in the process." – Dr. Kyle

The First Impression Formula:

Front Desk (30 seconds):

- Warm greeting using patient's first name
- "We're so excited to meet you today!"
- Immediate comfort establishment
- Clear explanation of what happens next

Treatment Coordinator (2 minutes):

- Personal connection building
- Anxiety reduction techniques
- Office tour with strategic stops
- Confidence-building statements about the doctor

Doctor Entrance (60 seconds):

- Confident, unhurried presence
- Genuine interest in the person, not just the teeth
- Personality calibration (adjust energy to match theirs)
- Permission-based interaction

The Connection Secret: Find one non-dental thing to connect on within the first 2 minutes. Sports, school, pets, hobbies, mutual acquaintances. People buy from people they like. More importantly, people buy from people who seem to like them.

P #4: THE PROGRAM

"Don't forget that this is likely the patient and/or parent's first time in an Orthodontic office." – Dr. Kyle

The Perfect Program Script: "Before we begin, let me explain exactly what we're going to do today. First, I'm going to take a look at [patient's name]'s teeth and bite. This won't take long. Then I'll share what I see and discuss whether treatment would be beneficial. After that, [TC's name] will answer any questions about scheduling, payment options, and insurance. The whole process takes about 5 minutes. Does that sound good?"

This approach reduces anxiety through predictability and positions you as organized and professional.

P #5: THE PROBLEM

"What is the patient's chief complaint? This is why they came and it's the most important part of the consultation." – Dr. Kyle

The $100,000 Question: "What brought you in to see us today?" Then STOP TALKING and listen.

The 3-Layer Problem Discovery:

1. **Surface Problem:** "Her teeth are crooked"

2. **Emotional Problem:** "She's embarrassed to smile"

3. **Future Problem:** "I'm worried it will affect her confidence in high school"

Perfect Problem Questions:

- "How long has this been bothering you?"

- "What made you decide to do something about it now?"

- "How do you think this affects [patient's name]?"

- "What would happen if we don't address this?"

- "How important is it to you that we fix this?"

P #6: THE PEEK

"Take a look at the patient's teeth. Even if you already know what you're going to do, you may have missed something." – Dr. Kyle

The Perfect Peek Protocol:

- Verbalize what you see: "I can see why this bothers you".

- Point out things they haven't noticed: "You may not have realized...".

- Use patient-friendly language: "crowding and an overbite" not "dental malocclusion and a class II bite".

- Take photos and show them immediately.
- Explain the progression: "This will only get worse over time".

P #7: THE PLAN

"Share your orthodontic treatment plan, how long you predict it will take, and what role the patient will need to play." – Dr. Kyle

The Perfect Plan Presentation:

1. **The Problem Recap:** "As we discussed, the main issues are..."
2. **The Solution Overview:** "Here's how we're going to transform your smile..."
3. **The Timeline:** "The process typically takes..."
4. **The Cooperation Required:** "Here's what I need from you..."
5. **The Outcome:** "When we're finished, you'll have..."

The Confidence Close: "I've treated over 2,000 patients with similar issues, and I'm confident we can give you an absolutely beautiful result."

P #8: THE PAUSE

"Give the patient and/or parent an opportunity to have a voice." – Dr. Kyle

After presenting your treatment plan, say: "What questions do you have?" Then count to 5 before speaking again.

The Objection Prevention Strategy: Address common concerns before they're raised:

- "Many parents wonder if their child is too young/old for treatment..."
- "Some people are concerned about the appearance of braces..."
- "I know cost is always a consideration..."

P #9: THE PASS OFF

"One of the most important steps in the Perfect Consult is to empower your TC to finish the job and make the sale." – Dr. Kyle

The Perfect Pass Off Script: "[TC's name] is our treatment coordinator and financial specialist. She's worked with me for [X years] and she's an expert at helping families get started with treatment. She'll go over the investment options and answer any questions about scheduling. She'll also take excellent care of you throughout the entire treatment process."

The Confidence Boost: Before leaving, make a statement that increases urgency and desire:

- "I'm really excited about your case. You're going to love your new smile."
- "This is exactly the type of transformation we specialize in."
- "I can't wait to see your reaction when we take your braces off."

P #10: THE PRAYER

"Upon leaving the exam room, I always say a silent prayer—that the patient starts OR that they don't start…" – Dr. Kyle

The Selection Process: Not every patient is right for your practice. The Prayer step is about quality control.

Red Flag Patients:

- Price shoppers (only care about cost)
- Compliance concerns (won't follow instructions)
- Unrealistic expectations (want perfection in 6 months)
- Difficult personalities (rude, demanding, argumentative)

The "No" Script: "After examining [patient's name], I'm concerned that I won't be able to make you completely happy with the results. I think you'd be better served by seeking another opinion."

Understand that some patients' needs, expectations, or values may not align with what your practice offers.

The Power of Assumptive Selling

Everything you say and do should point toward the next step in the process—not asking for it or speaking of it in a hypothetical way, but assuming it will happen.

Manifestation in this regard is incredibly powerful.

Instead of: "If you decide to move forward..." **Say:** "When we start your treatment next month..."

Instead of: "Would you be interested in scheduling?" **Say:** "Let's get you scheduled. What works better for you—mornings or afternoons?"

Instead of: "Do you have any questions about payment?" **Say:** "Which payment option works best for your family's budget?"

This linguistic shift creates psychological momentum. When you speak with certainty, patients feel the confidence they need to commit.

The Down Payment Reality Check

How can you ever know if patients are truly committed? Well, you can't exactly, but a reasonable threshold helps.

A reasonable approach includes:

- **Down payment of around $750** (demonstrates genuine commitment)
- **Monthly payments of around $200** (sustainable for most committed families)
- **Payment period that extends 6 months beyond the estimated length of treatment**

Example: On a 24-month case, with $200 monthly payments and a $750 down payment, that equates to 30 months and $6,750 of total expense—which should cover most cases while ensuring patient commitment.

This approach filters for patients who are genuinely committed to treatment completion and payment responsibility, rather than those attracted primarily by convenience.

Building Trust Through Ethical Sales Approaches

The word "sales" often triggers negative reactions in healthcare settings. Yet the most successful practices recognize that ethical persuasion is both necessary and beneficial—when it prioritizes patient well-being above all else.

Ethical sales in healthcare means aligning treatments with genuine patient needs and desires while building a sustainable practice model.

This starts with comprehensive discovery conversations where treatment coordinators explore personal goals as well as not just clinical conditions. What brings this patient to seek care? What outcomes matter most to them? How do they define success?

When patients sense you're more committed to their well-being than to selling a particular treatment, resistance naturally diminishes. Trust becomes the foundation of the relationship.

Measuring What Actually Matters

Stop obsessing over conversion rates in isolation. The metrics that actually drive practice success and life balance are:

1. **Revenue per lead:** Total revenue ÷ number of leads

2. **Profit per start:** After all expenses, what do you actually take home?

3. **Lifetime value realization:** Are you capturing retreatment and referral opportunities?

4. **Collection efficiency:** What percentage of committed revenue do you actually collect?

5. **Time to cash:** How quickly do payment commitments turn into received payments?

6. **Default rate:** What percentage of patients complete their payment obligations?

The Lead Value Calculation That Changes Everything

So, what's a lead worth? It depends. Let's work backwards...

3 Key Factors to Consider:

1. **Lifetime Value (LTV):** A patient's total value goes beyond the initial case. Retreatment (1 in 40 patients) and purchases like replacement retainers ($500 on average) add up significantly over time.

2. **Referrals:** A happy patient who refers others adds even more value—with no extra marketing cost.

3. **Conversion Rate:** Not every lead becomes a patient. In orthodontics, the average conversion rate is about 70%.

How to Calculate Lead Value: Multiply LTV by your conversion rate. For example: $6,680 LTV × 70% conversion = $4,676 per lead.

Remember the $4,700 exercise? Run this scenario with your entire team regularly. When everyone understands that each patient interaction carries that same value, behaviors change immediately.

So, the first thing you do is understand the value of a lead. Then:

1. **Decide how much you want to spend and where:** How much are you willing to invest in marketing, and where do you want to spend it? Pick options that deliver the most profitable results.

2. **Optimize your Sales and Admin Systems:** Revisit and improve your treatment coordination processes.

3. **Measure ROI:** Do the math on every marketing effort. Count the new patients, calculate their treatment value, subtract your costs. Then make the obvious choice: invest more in what works, stop funding what doesn't.

4. **Repeat:** Do it over and over, refining the process along the way so that it continuously improves.

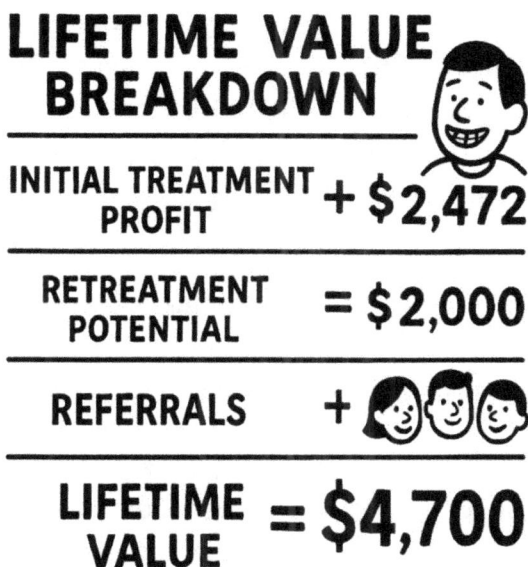

LIFETIME VALUE BREAKDOWN

INITIAL TREATMENT PROFIT	+ $2,472
RETREATMENT POTENTIAL	= $2,000
REFERRALS	+ 🙂🙂🙂
LIFETIME VALUE	= $4,700

The Practice Paradox Resolved

Mastering the treatment coordination process transforms not just your practice's financial health but your entire relationship with your profession. The strategies we've discussed allow you to create alignment between what patients truly need, what your practice can sustainably deliver, and the life you want to live.

When your treatment coordinators employ the ethical approaches outlined in this chapter, something remarkable happens. Patients no longer feel "sold to" but rather guided through options that genuinely address their concerns while supporting your practice's sustainability.

The art of treatment coordination, when mastered, allows you to build the practice of your dreams while helping patients achieve optimal health outcomes. This balance doesn't happen by accident—it requires intention, training, and consistent refinement.

Take time this week to assess your current treatment coordination protocols. Look for gaps between your ideal process and daily reality. Calculate your true lead value. Evaluate whether your metrics are driving the right behaviors.

Remember: your practice should serve your life, not consume it. When treatment coordination is done right, it creates the financial foundation that supports both excellent patient care and the work-life integration you deserve.

The choice is yours: continue chasing conversion rates that don't translate to sustainable success, or build a system that attracts, converts, and retains patients who value what you offer while supporting the lifestyle you've worked so hard to create.

Your $4,700 opportunity walks through your door with every new patient. Make it count.

Key Takeaways

- Conversion rate is a vanity metric; what matters most is profit per patient and lifetime value.
- Each qualified lead is worth ~$4,700 in profit. Treat them accordingly.
- High acceptance rates achieved through discounts and insurance participation often erode profitability and increase burnout.
- Treatment coordination works best when driven by trained treatment coordinators, not only the doctor.
- The Perfect Consult™ framework provides a proven, repeatable system for building trust and increasing case acceptance.
- Ethical sales is not manipulation. It is guiding patients toward the care they need while ensuring the sustainability of your practice.

Next Steps

You don't have to overhaul your entire consultation system to see results. Starting this week, you can:

Calculate the lifetime value of a patient – Include retreatment, retainers, and referrals in your math.

Reassess your current consultation process – Identify where delays, dead time, or overemphasis on conversion rates may be costing you money.

Empower your treatment coordinator – Allow them to guide patients through financial discussions to maintain momentum and increase starts.

When you master treatment coordination, you don't just get more patients, you get the right patients saying yes. But yes is only the beginning. Those patients expect the service and results you've promised, and you can't deliver that by carrying the whole load yourself. Grip too tightly, and you end up back in the practice paradox.

The way forward is to empower your team. Train them to think like orthodontists, give them systems that make excellence predictable, and free yourself from being the bottleneck. That's what the next chapter is all about—clinical implementation done right.

Chapter 9: Clinical Implementation Excellence

By: Dr. Kyle Fagala

Dr. Rachel stood at her kitchen counter, planner open, staring at two columns she'd drawn: work on the left, family on the right. On paper, the practice was thriving—patient load was up, collections were steady, and the reputation was strong. But every day felt like a grind of micromanagement, endless oversight, and missed moments with her family. She knew her assistants were capable, but she couldn't let go. Every clinical decision and task still seemed to flow through her. And the more she tried to control every detail, the less control she actually felt.

That's the paradox at the heart of clinical implementation: the tighter you grip, the more fragile your practice becomes. True excellence doesn't come from doing everything yourself. It comes from building systems, protocols, and empowered teams that deliver consistently, whether you're in the room or not. When you shift from control to orchestration, you reclaim both clinical excellence and personal freedom.

This chapter is about Clinical Implementation Excellence. The discipline of designing workflows, training your team, and simplifying protocols so your practice runs at a high standard every day without burning you out. We'll explore how to structure roles, empower assistants to think like clinicians, streamline your systems for consistency, and maintain quality as a non-negotiable standard. Done right, implementation turns chaos into choreography and restores the joy that drew you into practice in the first place.

The Control Paradox

Here's an insight that can transform your practice: **the tighter you grip control over every clinical detail, the more control actually slips through your fingers.**

We've been conditioned to believe that quality care requires our personal involvement in every decision, every procedure, every patient interaction. This thinking creates practices where excellence depends entirely on the doctor's presence—fragile systems that crumble the moment you step away.

The practice paradox reveals itself most clearly in clinical implementation: true mastery comes from building systems that work without you, not systems that depend on you.

The orthodontists and dentists who achieve both exceptional results and personal freedom have learned to leverage their expertise through systems, protocols, and trained team members. They've discovered that **delegating clinical responsibilities—when done correctly—often produces more consistent outcomes than trying to do everything themselves.**

Many practice owners find themselves trapped in a cycle of micromanagement and perfectionism. They believe only they can perform certain tasks correctly, leading to exhaustion and preventing team members from developing their full capabilities. This approach creates a bottleneck where quality care depends entirely on the doctor's direct involvement. The result? Burnout becomes inevitable, staff feel undervalued, and patients experience the downstream effects of an overtaxed system. The practice that was built to help others becomes the very thing harming its founder.

The relationship between workplace fulfillment and practice success represents the central paradox we've been exploring throughout this book. When clinicians prioritize creating environments where people genuinely want to work, financial success follows naturally. The inverse approach—chasing profits while neglecting culture—typically produces neither happiness nor sustainable growth.

When the Joy Seeps Out

The coffee finished brewing as Dr. Rachel flipped through her planner again, her eyes lingering on the long list of patients stacked back-to-back. Yesterday's staff meeting echoed in her mind—Melissa admitting she felt stretched too thin, Jack pointing out that small mistakes were starting to creep in, even among the most reliable assistants. It wasn't incompetence. It was pressure she had created by refusing to loosen her grip.

She caught herself remembering Emma's disappointed expression after the missed championship game. That memory hurt more than any difficult day at the office. In that moment, Rachel realized the cost of trying to control everything wasn't just her team's burnout. It was her own family's fading trust.

As the toast grew cold on her plate, she understood that her problem wasn't time management; it was trust management. Her team had the skills. What they lacked was the authority to truly own their roles. If she could build systems that empowered them to act without her constant oversight, she could reclaim more than just efficiency. She could reclaim her life.

That morning, Rachel made a decision. She would stop measuring her worth by how many tasks she completed personally, and start measuring it by how well her practice functioned without her. That shift, letting go of control to build stronger systems, was the key to both clinical excellence and the freedom she longed for.

The Kitchen That Changed Everything

Standing in your practice at 2:47 PM on a chaotic Tuesday, you realize something's fundamentally broken. Three assistants scramble between operatories, patients wait beyond their scheduled times, and you feel like a short-order cook trying to manage every order simultaneously.

Then you remember that dinner at Le Bernardin. Not just the exquisite food, but the seamless choreography of the kitchen. Executive Chef Eric Ripert orchestrated from the pass, the expeditor coordinated timing and quality, and the line cooks executed with precision. No wasted motion. No confusion about roles. Just efficient excellence that made the impossible look effortless.

Chef Ripert didn't cook every dish personally. Instead, he designed systems, trained his team, and maintained quality standards. **He understood that his highest value wasn't in performing every task but in ensuring every task was performed correctly.**

Your practice needs this same structure:

- **Executive Chef (You):** Sets standards, makes complex decisions, handles cases only you can handle

- **Expeditor (Clinical Coordinator):** Ensures quality, coordinates flow, troubleshoots problems, maintains standards

- **Line Cooks (Clinical Assistants):** Execute protocols, prepare patients, handle routine procedures with expertise

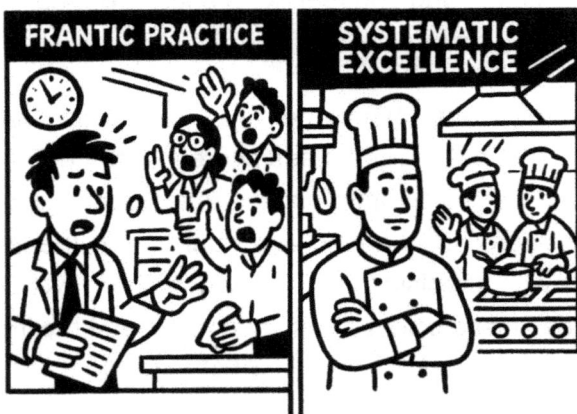

IS YOUR PRACTICE A SHORT-ORDER KITCHEN OR A FINE-DINING OPERATION?

FRANTIC PRACTICE

SYSTEMATIC EXCELLENCE

The Clinical Coordinator: Your Practice Expeditor

The clinical coordinator role transforms everything. This person isn't tied to a specific chair but rather moves throughout the practice ensuring that your clinical vision is executed consistently across every patient interaction. **They become your eyes and ears, catching problems before they become crises and ensuring seamless patient flow.**

Instead of you running between rooms putting out fires, someone else maintains orchestration while you focus on clinical decisions that truly require your expertise. They make sure wires are ready, chairs are prepared, supplies are stocked, and each patient's care follows established protocols. When a patient runs late, they adjust the schedule. When an assistant has a question, they provide guidance or escalate appropriately. When equipment malfunctions, they handle the solution.

This role is about multiplying effectiveness. A skilled clinical coordinator enables your other team members to work at the top of their capabilities while making sure nothing falls through the cracks. **They become the conductor of your clinical orchestra, allowing you to be the virtuoso performer you trained to be.**

The investment in this role pays for itself through improved efficiency, reduced stress, and enhanced patient experience. More importantly, it gives you back the joy of practicing orthodontics without drowning in the minutiae of daily operations. You reclaim mental bandwidth for the complex clinical decisions that genuinely require your expertise.

Consider the ripple effects: when your clinical coordinator handles routine coordination, your assistants can focus on patient care rather than logistics. When assistants aren't distracted by organizational concerns, they provide better chairside assistance. When you're not constantly interrupted by operational issues, you can give full attention to each patient. **Everyone operates at their highest level of capability.**

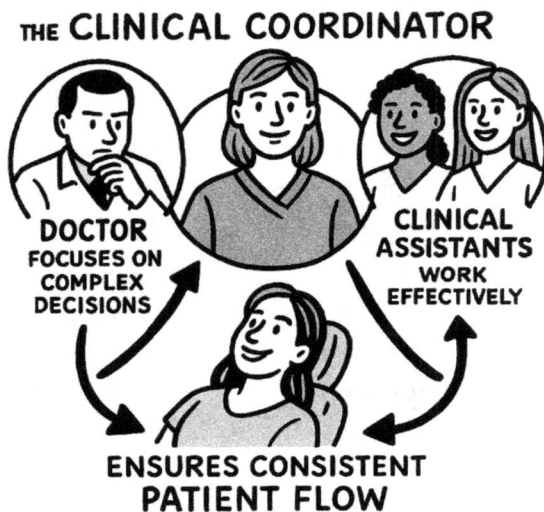

THE **CLINICAL COORDINATOR**

DOCTOR
FOCUSES ON
COMPLEX
DECISIONS

**CLINICAL
ASSISTANTS**
WORK
EFFECTIVELY

**ENSURES CONSISTENT
PATIENT FLOW**

Creating Consistent Clinical Excellence Through Systems

Clinical consistency doesn't happen by accident. **It requires intentional design and implementation of systems that work for your team and patients.** Streamlined processes reduce errors, save time, and create a sense of order that benefits everyone in your practice.

Think again of your clinical workflows like the kitchen of a fine restaurant. Each chef knows exactly where tools are stored, when to start each component of a dish, and how to plate the final creation. This orchestrated dance allows for consistent quality no matter who's cooking that night. **Similarly, well-designed clinical processes ensure patients receive the same high-quality care regardless of which team member assists them or what day they visit.**

Inconsistency creates friction at every level. When staff members perform the same task differently, it leads to confusion, wasted time, and frustration. Patients notice these variations too—whether it's inconsistent communication about treatment plans, different approaches to scheduling follow-ups, or varying levels of attention to comfort measures. These small discrepancies erode trust and undermine your practice's professional image.

The Foundation of Systematic Excellence

Efficiency doesn't mean rushing through appointments. Rather, it means eliminating unnecessary steps and streamlining necessary ones so you can focus more time on actual patient care. Start by mapping your current clinical processes from check-in to check-out. Follow a typical patient's journey through your practice and identify every touchpoint, every handoff, every potential delay.

Ask yourself: Where do bottlenecks occur? What steps could be simplified or eliminated? Where do team members seem confused about procedures? What questions get asked repeatedly? **These observations reveal opportunities for systematic improvement.**

Documentation plays a crucial role in clinical consistency. Create clear, accessible protocols for common procedures, from patient intake to treatment delivery. **These should be living documents, regularly reviewed and updated based on team feedback and evolving best practices.**

But documentation alone isn't enough. **The protocols must be practical, easily referenced during busy periods, and designed with input from the people who will actually use them.** A protocol that looks perfect on paper but proves cumbersome in practice will be ignored when schedules get tight.

Small changes often yield significant results. Something as simple as standardizing how exam rooms are stocked and organized can save minutes per appointment—minutes that add up to hours over weeks and months. **These reclaimed moments create space for more meaningful patient interactions or allow you to maintain a schedule that respects everyone's time.**

The goal is predictability. When your team knows what to expect and how to respond to common situations, they operate with confidence rather than anxiety. This confidence translates into better patient care and a more enjoyable work environment for everyone involved.

Training Clinical Decision-Makers

Here's a thought experiment that will change how you think about delegation: spend a day with your hands tied behind your back. How much of your job could you still accomplish?

The answer reveals how much of your current work doesn't actually require your direct physical involvement. Specific to Orthodontics, your clinical assistants can evaluate cases, develop daily treatment plans, write preliminary notes, and make informed recommendations—if they're trained properly.

The traditional model treats assistants as task-followers who implement your instructions without deeper understanding. This approach wastes their intellectual capacity and keeps you trapped in micromanagement.

Instead of training assistants to follow simple protocols, train them to think like orthodontists.

The Evaluation Revolution

When you arrive at each chair, rather than starting from scratch with basic assessment, you should be reviewing recommendations and confirming treatment plans developed by properly trained team members. This fundamental shift provides multiple benefits:

- **Efficiency:** Your time focuses on clinical decisions rather than data gathering. Instead of spending five minutes evaluating what's obvious, you spend two minutes confirming recommendations and addressing complex issues.

- **Quality:** Two sets of eyes improve accuracy and catch potential issues before they become problems. Your assistant's fresh perspective might notice something you missed or raise questions that lead to better treatment decisions.

- **Development:** Team members gain skills and job satisfaction through expanded responsibilities. They develop genuine expertise rather than just following rote procedures.

- **Flow:** Appointments progress faster and more smoothly when proper preparation occurs before your arrival. Patients receive more attention because time isn't wasted on basic data gathering.

The Systematic Evaluation Protocol

While these protocols can be adapted for any dental specialty, here's how to train orthodontic assistants in a comprehensive evaluation process:

1. **Review Current Status:** Assess progress, cooperation, hygiene, and appliance condition since the last visit.

2. **Appliance Assessment:** Check bracket integrity, wire condition, and elastic wear. Document any issues requiring attention.

3. **Progress Evaluation:** Compare current positions to treatment goals and note any movement concerns.

4. **Issue Identification:** Flag problems like poor hygiene, broken appliances, or lack of cooperation.

5. **Protocol Application:** Recommend next steps—wire changes, elastic adjustments, or appointment intervals.

6. **Documentation:** Prepare preliminary notes summarizing findings and recommendations.

7. **Presentation:** Present findings clearly upon doctor's arrival, highlighting concerns or deviations from expected progress.

This doesn't mean assistants make final clinical decisions—they gather information, apply established protocols, and make informed recommendations within their scope of training. You maintain ultimate authority while benefiting from their preparation and observations.

SYSTEMATIC EVALUATION PROTOCOL

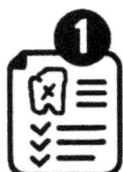

1 ### REVIEW CURRENT STATUS
Assess progress, cooperation, hygiene, and appliance condition since the last visit.

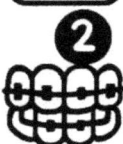

2 ### APPLIANCE ASSESSMENT
Check bracket integrity, wire condition, and elastic wear. Document any issues.

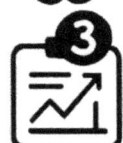

3 ### PROGRESS EVALUATION
Compare current positions to treatment goals and note movement concerns.

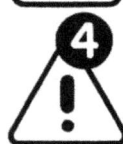

4 ### ISSUE IDENTIFICATION
Flag problems like poor hygiene, broken appliances, or lack of cooperation.

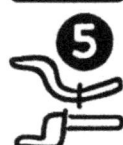

5 ### PROTOCOL APPLICATION
Recommend next steps – wire changes, elastic adjustments, or appointment intervals

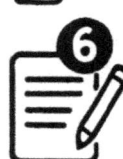

6 ### DOCUMENTATION
Prepare preliminary notes summarizing findings and recommendations.

7 ### PRESENTATION
Present findings clearly upon doctor's arrival

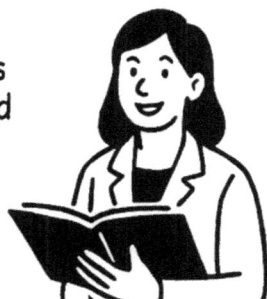

The Power of Systematic Simplification

Complexity is the enemy of consistency. The more variables you introduce into your clinical protocols, the more decisions you create, and the more opportunities for confusion arise. Every additional option multiplies the mental load on both you and your team, creating decision fatigue that slows progress and introduces errors.

The most successful dentists and orthodontists have learned to limit themselves to core sequences and protocols for the vast majority of cases, reserving specialty approaches for specific situations that truly require them.

Take wire progressions, for example. Rather than having dozens of wire options creating constant decision points, develop a streamlined sequence that handles 95% of your cases predictably. Reserve specialty wires only for cases that truly require their unique properties.

The same principle applies to every aspect of clinical care: appointment scheduling, treatment planning protocols, finishing procedures, and patient communication. **Simplification means creating clarity that enables quality to emerge more consistently without compromising quality.**

The Benefits of Systematic Thinking

When you limit yourself to proven, systematic approaches, several things happen:

For You: Fewer decisions reduce mental fatigue and speed treatment planning. Predictable timelines make scheduling easier and patient communication clearer. Treatment becomes more systematic and less stressful.

For Your Team: Clear protocols eliminate confusion about what comes next. Consistent inventory management reduces complexity and ordering errors. Simplified scheduling makes appointment planning straightforward.

For Patients: More predictable appointments create realistic expectations. Clearer treatment progression improves compliance. Better communication about treatment phases increases satisfaction.

Never Compromise on Clinical Results

Here's a hard truth that transcends all other considerations: no amount of customer service, communication skills, operational efficiency, or marketing sophistication can compensate for consistently poor clinical results.

Patients might forgive a scheduling mishap, understand communication breakdowns, or tolerate occasional inconveniences. **But they will not forgive teeth that don't look right or function properly when treatment ends.** They will not refer friends and family if their own results are mediocre. They will not provide positive reviews if their smiles didn't meet expectations.

Your clinical reputation is everything. It determines referrals, online reviews, team morale, personal satisfaction, and ultimately the sustainability of your practice. Every case that leaves your office either enhances or diminishes that reputation. There's no middle ground, no neutral outcomes. Each patient becomes either an advocate or a cautionary tale.

The Excellence Standard

Commit to showing up every day willing to work hard for exceptional results. This commitment requires discipline, especially when external pressures mount:

- **Never settle for "good enough" when you know better is possible.** The temptation to accept compromised solutions grows stronger when schedules are tight, but these decisions compound over time to damage your reputation.

- **Take the time required for proper finishing, even when efficiency pressures build.** The extra appointment or additional month of treatment that achieves ideal results pays dividends for years through referrals and reputation enhancement. It's also the right thing to do.

- **Stay current with techniques and technologies that improve outcomes.** Clinical excellence requires continuous learning and adaptation as new methods prove superior to traditional approaches.

- **Seek consultation for complex cases rather than struggling alone.** Recognizing the limits of your expertise and consulting with specialists or colleagues demonstrates professional maturity and protects patient outcomes.

- **Maintain standards even when external pressures mount.** Economic pressures, schedule demands, or patient requests should never compromise your clinical standards.

The Long-Term Perspective

Think beyond today's schedule to next year's reputation. The patient you rush through today to maintain efficiency might become the poor result that haunts your practice for years. Conversely, the extra time invested in achieving an exceptional outcome often generates referrals that more than compensate for short-term efficiency sacrifices.

Consider the mathematics of reputation: one outstanding result might generate five new patients through referrals over two years. One poor result might cost you ten potential patients who choose other providers based on negative reviews or word-of-mouth reports. The economic incentives strongly favor clinical excellence, even when it requires short-term sacrifices.

Patient expectations have evolved significantly. Social media, before-and-after galleries, and increased awareness of orthodontic outcomes mean **patients expect exceptional results, not just improved teeth.** Meeting these elevated expectations requires commitment to true excellence rather than adequate improvement.

The Business Case for Excellence

Exceptional clinical results are ethically correct—but they also represent smart business strategy. **Patients with outstanding results become your most effective marketing asset.** They refer friends, leave positive reviews, provide testimonials, and serve as walking advertisements for your practice.

The practice built on clinical excellence operates from a position of strength. You compete on results rather than price, attract patients who value quality, and build a reputation that sustains long-term growth. Premium positioning becomes possible when outcomes justify premium fees.

Team morale improves dramatically when clinical results are consistently excellent. Team members take pride in being associated with exceptional outcomes, leading to better retention, increased referrals from staff, and higher performance standards throughout the practice.

Your own job satisfaction increases immeasurably when results consistently meet your standards. The stress of managing poor outcomes, difficult conversations, and reputation damage disappears when clinical excellence becomes your standard operating procedure.

Implementation: Building Your Clinical Excellence Foundation

Don't attempt to transform everything simultaneously. Clinical excellence is built through consistent improvement over time, not dramatic overnight changes. Start with one area where improvement would yield the greatest impact and build systematically from there.

Week 1-2: Assessment and Planning

Evaluate your current patient flow and identify the primary bottleneck limiting your efficiency or quality. This might be preparation delays, unclear protocols, inadequate delegation, or finishing inconsistencies.

Week 3-4: Clinical Coordination

Train one experienced team member as a clinical coordinator. Start with basic responsibilities and gradually expand their role as competency develops.

Week 5-6: Protocol Simplification

Standardize your approach to core clinical procedures. Document the protocols and train your team on simplified, consistent sequences.

Week 7-8: Quality Systems

Establish checkpoints and evaluation systems that maintain standards without micromanagement. Create feedback loops that enable continuous improvement.

Communication proves essential during this transformation process. Your team needs to understand not just what changes are being made but why they matter for patient care, practice efficiency, and job satisfaction. Connect improvements to meaningful outcomes like reduced stress, enhanced patient experience, and more predictable schedules.

The implementation process will reveal where your leadership is most needed. Some team members will enthusiastically embrace new protocols and expanded responsibilities. Others may resist change or struggle with new expectations. **Your consistent reinforcement of standards, investment in training, and recognition of progress will determine whether changes become permanent improvements.**

The Clinical Paradox Resolved

When all these elements work together—clinical coordination, refined techniques, optimized flow, simplified systems, and unwavering quality standards—something remarkable happens. **Your practice transforms into an orchestra where every member knows their part, timing becomes effortless, and the result is beautiful music.**

The morning huddle sets a productive tone with clear communication and preparation. Each team member understands their role and responsibilities. Clinical progressions follow predictable sequences that everyone understands. Quality checkpoints maintain standards throughout treatment without creating bureaucratic burden.

The result? Days that feel manageable rather than overwhelming, team members who take pride in their expanding capabilities, and clinical results that consistently exceed both your standards and patient expectations.

This represents the practice paradox resolved: exceptional care and operational joy are complementary forces that reinforce each other. The practice that operates efficiently creates more time for quality care. The practice that consistently delivers quality care attracts patients who appreciate excellence and generates the referrals that sustain growth.

By integrating streamlined processes, strategic delegation, and reliable protocols through systematic implementation,

you create a practice where clinical excellence becomes the natural outcome rather than a constant struggle.

The Joy of True Mastery

When clinical systems operate smoothly, something wonderful happens: you rediscover why you became an orthodontist or dentist. Instead of fighting administrative battles and operational fires all day, you focus on the intellectually stimulating aspects of diagnosis, treatment planning, and complex problem-solving that drew you to the profession originally.

Your days become more predictable and more satisfying. The chaos that once characterized busy periods gives way to orchestrated efficiency. **Patients receive better care because you have more mental bandwidth for their individual needs. Team members develop genuine expertise and pride in their expanding capabilities, becoming true partners in delivering excellence rather than task-followers waiting for instructions.**

The transformation affects every aspect of your practice experience. Mornings begin with purposeful preparation rather than frantic catch-up. Patient interactions become more meaningful because systems handle the routine aspects efficiently. Lunch breaks become actual breaks rather than administrative catch-up time. Evenings end with satisfaction rather than exhaustion.

Most importantly, you reclaim ownership of your professional identity. Instead of feeling controlled by your practice's demands, you actively shape how care is delivered. Instead of reacting to daily crises, you proactively design systems that prevent problems. Instead of working harder to achieve the same results, you work more intelligently to achieve better outcomes with greater satisfaction.

Moving Forward: Your Implementation Journey

The journey toward implementation excellence is ongoing, and it requires continuous attention to systems, commitment to standards, and willingness to adapt as circumstances change. But the framework provides the structure for sustainable progress rather than endless reinvention.

Start where you are, with what you have, addressing the most pressing needs first. Build systematically rather than dramatically. Measure progress rather than pursuing perfection. Celebrate improvements rather than focusing only on remaining challenges.

As you move forward, keep asking the question that drives all meaningful progress: **"How can we make this better while making our lives better?"** That question—perhaps more than any specific protocol or system—will guide you toward the practice of your dreams.

The greatest achievement isn't building a practice that impresses others with its sophistication or efficiency. It's building one that allows you and your team to do your best work while living your best lives. A practice that challenges you to grow while supporting your wellbeing. A business that generates success while preserving the values that made you choose healthcare as your calling.

The practice of your dreams is waiting to be built. Implementation excellence is how you build it.

Key Takeaways

- Micromanagement creates fragility. Systems and empowered teams create strength.

- Clinical coordinators and clear protocols turn chaos into choreography.

- Training assistants to think like clinicians improves efficiency, quality, and satisfaction.

- Simplification is the key to consistency. Limit unnecessary complexity.

- Clinical excellence is non-negotiable. It drives reputation, referrals, and long-term success.

Next Steps

You don't need to overhaul your practice overnight. Starting this week, you can:

Identify one bottleneck – Map your patient flow and choose one area to simplify.

Clarify a protocol – Document and train your team on a single core process.

Empower one team member – Give an assistant or coordinator responsibility and authority over a specific clinical area.

Set a quality checkpoint – Add one step in your process where standards are verified before moving forward.

By now, you've seen how the right systems, empowered teams, and consistent clinical excellence can free you from the practice paradox and give you back control. But there's a hidden truth most doctors ignore: none of it works if you, the leader, the clinician, the driving force, are running on empty.

That's why your most valuable asset isn't your team, your technology, or even your clinical expertise. It's you. In the next chapter, we'll show you why investing in your health is the ultimate lever for sustaining the freedom, joy, and profitability you've been building and how to create routines that make your career (and your life outside of it) not just sustainable, but fulfilling.

Section V: Life Beyond the Clinic

Discover:

Chapter 10 – Your Most Valuable Asset: Why your health is the foundation of your professional and personal success.

Chapter 11 – Entrepreneurial Opportunities and Passive Income: How building revenue streams beyond the chair creates freedom and long-term security.

Chapter 10: Your Most Valuable Asset

By: Luke Infinger

Dr. Bill sat in his darkened office long after the last patient had left, staring at the glow of his computer screen. The day's numbers looked good—full schedule, solid production, collections on track. But he didn't feel good. He hadn't for months. Skipping breakfast, running on caffeine, wolfing down a sandwich at lunch, and pushing through back-to-back procedures had left him drained. His body ached, his patience was thin, and even his family barely saw him anymore. On paper, everything was fine. But he wasn't.

Bill had fallen into the trap too many doctors face—sacrificing his health for his practice, only to realize the practice was consuming him.

This chapter explores the direct link between your personal health and your professional success. We'll look at the risks of neglecting your wellbeing, the practices and protocols that high-performing clinicians use to stay sharp, and the mindset shifts that connect your health to your purpose. From nutrition and recovery to mindfulness and energy management, you'll learn how to build a health operating system that keeps you in your performance zone for decades, not just years. Because your patients, your team, and your family don't need a burned-out doctor. They need the best version of you.

Why Your Health Determines Your Success

"A sick person has only one wish, but a healthy person has a thousand wishes."

The tension between excelling at your craft and keeping your sanity is universal. I've seen countless talented clinicians sacrifice their health, their families, and their joy on the altar of "success." The cruel irony is that sacrifice almost never delivers what they thought it would.

The bridge between burnout and balance is simpler than most realize: **strategic delegation.**

But here's the problem—most clinicians completely misunderstand what real delegation is. They think it's about dumping tasks to lighten their load. At best, it feels like a shortcut. At worst, it feels like giving up control.

They're wrong.

True delegation is leadership. Done right, it changes your culture, grows your team, and creates space for you to focus on what really matters—at work and at home. In my experience, it's the single most powerful lever for reclaiming your time, your energy, and your sanity.

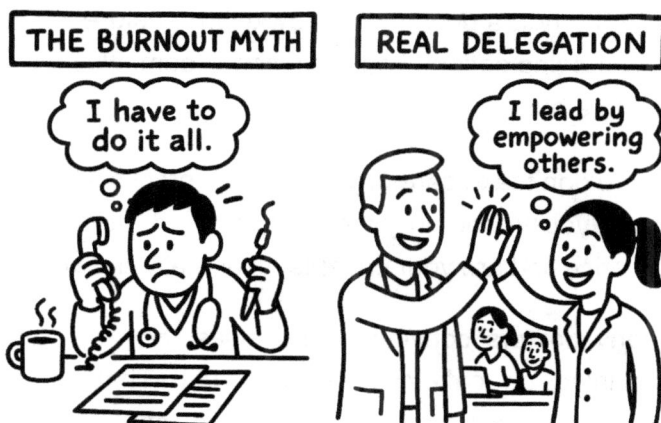

The data backs it up: dentists who master delegation report 43% higher job satisfaction and 37% lower burnout than those who try to do it all themselves. Not because they're working less—but because they're finally working on the right things.

When you delegate well, you'll realize that you actually gain authority. You empower your team, and they step up. Patients notice the difference. And you finally have the bandwidth to make the high-level decisions that actually move the needle.

This is the ripple effect no one talks about: delegation builds trust. It creates growth. It makes your practice more efficient, more profitable, and a better place for everyone to show up every day—including you.

The Missing Link Between Practice and Personal Health

You might not realize it, but your personal health drives your practice. The demands of orthodontics and dentistry are unique: long hours on your feet, awkward postures, constant focus, managing patients, parents, and a team, plus the stress of running a business.

When you don't take care of yourself, the cracks show in your energy, in your mood, in your patience. And the people who pay the price first are your patients, your staff, and your family.

Too many doctors convince themselves they can "tough it out," running on caffeine and willpower. That works—for a while. But it's a losing game. Burnout, chronic pain, and disengagement are what's waiting at the finish line.

Taking care of yourself isn't indulgent. It's your professional obligation. Your practice needs you to show up sharp, calm, and focused every day. That means building habits that protect your body, sharpen your mind, and help you recover from the grind of clinical life.

The Burden of Trust

Dr. Bill rubbed his temples and thought back to the conversation with his doctor last month: *"Your blood work looks normal... maybe you're just stressed."* Normal didn't feel this bad. Normal didn't explain the brain fog, the short temper with staff, the constant ache in his shoulders, or the fact that he couldn't remember the last dinner he'd made it home for.

That night, as he sat alone in the office, a memory surfaced. During residency, one of his mentors had told him: *"Your patients will always take as much as you're willing to give. But you only have so much to give if you don't refill your own tank."*

For the first time, he wondered what it would look like to take that seriously.

What if he stopped accepting "fine" as enough and started investigating why his body felt broken? What if he treated his own health with the same diligence he gave to his patients' care—comprehensive tests, root-cause solutions, not just patching symptoms with coffee and ibuprofen?

He pulled a notepad from his drawer and wrote down simple commitments:

- Book an appointment with a doctor who would dig deeper than "normal" blood-work.
- Replace caffeine and skipped meals with food that fueled him.
- Block time for movement, even short walks, instead of collapsing into his chair between patients.
- Try recovery tools he'd been hearing colleagues rave about—sauna, stretching, even cold plunges.
- Be home for dinner tomorrow.

As the list grew, something shifted. The heaviness he'd carried for months didn't disappear, but it lifted just enough to remind him that change was possible.

Bill realized his problem wasn't just physical. It was purpose. He had been showing up, producing, and providing but not pursuing anything bigger than the grind. Reconnecting to his "why" wasn't a luxury. It was the fuel he needed to keep going.

For the first time in a long time, he left the office with more than exhaustion. He left with resolve.

THE TURNING POINT

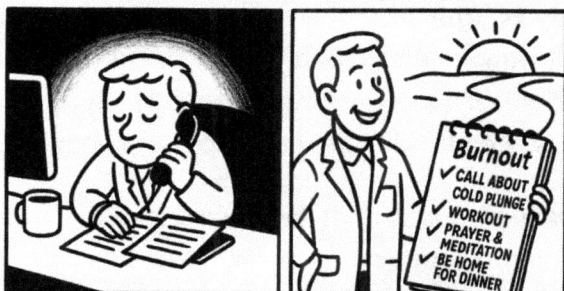

BURNOUT   **RESOLVE**

The Foundation of Professional Excellence

The connection between your personal health and your professional performance is physiological.

Your body is your practice's most important instrument. Every adjustment you make, every diagnosis you deliver, every patient you connect with depends on your ability to bring focus, steadiness, and presence into the room.

Yet too many clinicians treat their own bodies like a disposable tool—running on caffeine, skipping meals, cutting sleep, and letting stress silently accumulate. Then they wonder why their hands ache, their minds fog, their patience wears thin, and their passion fades.

It doesn't have to be this way.

When you fuel yourself properly with real food, restorative sleep, purposeful movement, and stress management, your brain fires sharper. Your creativity returns. Your endurance improves. Even your posture and fine motor control, both critical in this field, stay strong and steady under long hours.

The numbers back it up. A study in *Journal of Occupational Health Psychology* found that healthcare professionals who prioritized their health reported 27% higher job satisfaction and 31% lower burnout rates. ADA research showed that dentists who exercised regularly suffered 41% fewer muscu-loskeletal injuries—one of the most common reasons den-tists retire early.

And your patients can feel the difference, too. Whether consciously or not, people pick up on your energy, your mood, your clarity. **A provider who looks sharp, moves with confidence, and radiates calm inspires trust.** A provider who's visibly tired and impatient sends the opposite signal, no matter how clinically skilled they are.

Here's the hard truth: when you neglect your own health, you don't just pay the price yourself—your patients, your team, and your family feel it too.

Poor nutrition, chronic stress, and sleep deprivation set off an inflammatory cascade in the body. That shows up as aches and pains, slower reflexes, brain fog, irritability, even depression. Over time, this creates a vicious cycle: worse health leads to worse performance, which creates more stress, which further damages your health.

Breaking that cycle starts by respecting your body as your most valuable asset.

You'd never run a high-performance car on bad fuel and bald tires and expect it to keep winning races. Why treat yourself any differently?

No amount of CE courses or cutting-edge equipment can compensate for a provider who's running on fumes. If you want to deliver exceptional care, lead your team effectively, and still have energy left for your family at the end of the day, it starts here:

Take care of the one thing your practice can't function without—you.

Designing Your Health Operating System

If you want your career to last and your life outside it to feel meaningful, you need an operating system for your own health.

Too many doctors run on willpower and caffeine, patching together shortcuts like meds, fast food, and bad sleep. That's not sustainable. What you save in the short term shows up later as "health debt" in the form of stress hormones, inflammation, aches and pains, and burnout. You'd never tolerate sloppy systems in your practice. Why tolerate them in your own life?

Your body and mind are the infrastructure your practice runs on. Treat them like it.

Start with Nutrition

Precision work demands stable blood sugar, mental clarity, and energy. The "Standard American Diet" does the opposite.

Ditch the processed carbs and sugar. Build meals around high-protein, nutrient-dense, real food. Many high-performing clinicians thrive on Paleo, Carnivore, or at least a whole-food, high-protein approach. Why? Because it works—less inflammation, steadier energy, better focus. Keep clean snacks at the office. Eat like your livelihood depends on it, because it does.

Master Recovery

You can't "out-grind" chronic stress. Long days in awkward positions wreck your neck, back, and joints over time. Bake in proactive recovery: daily mobility, targeted stretching, massage, ergonomic habits. Sauna, cold plunge, red light therapy—these "biohacks" combat inflammation, improve circulation, and reset stress hormones. A 3-minute cold plunge can wake up your nervous system better than another espresso. A sauna session post-work helps you sleep like a rock. You don't have to do everything—but you can choose a couple tools that fit.

Movement Matters

You don't need an hour at the gym to stay fit. High-intensity intervals or resistance training 2–3 times a week can maintain the core strength and mobility your work demands. On busy days, sprinkle in "movement snacks"—push-ups, squats, stretches—between patients. Every little bit adds up.

Sleep is Non-Negotiable

No single change improves performance faster than getting consistent, high-quality rest. Fix your sleep environment: cool room, no screens late at night, consistent bedtime. The difference shows up the next morning in your mood, focus, and steadiness.

Leverage Technology

Wearables that track your sleep, HRV, and stress give you feedback to improve. Apps can guide breathwork or meditation to calm your mind. Meal prep services can keep you eating clean even during your busiest weeks. Use technology to support your body, not sabotage it.

The Purpose Element

But the most overlooked element of a health operating system isn't physical at all—it's **purpose.**

Studies show that people who find deep meaning in their work are happier, healthier, and more resilient. Your mindset—the reason you show up every day—fuels everything else. When you believe what you're doing matters, your body responds: lower stress, higher motivation, more grit. A wandering mind, by contrast, breeds unhappiness. So ask yourself regularly: *Why am I doing this? Who benefits from my best work?*

Doctors who build their routines around that sense of purpose and pair it with strategic nutrition, movement, recovery, and biohacks find that they perform better, lead better, and live better.

You wouldn't let your practice run without maintenance, calibration, and upgrades. Don't let your body and mind operate on autopilot, either. Build a system. Stick to it. Adjust as needed.

Your career—and the people who count on you—will thank you for it.

Mental Resilience in a High-Pressure Practice

Orthodontics may not feel dramatic on the surface, but it is relentless. Dozens of patients in a day, hundreds of small decisions, endless questions from patients, parents, and team members. Even in a calm, competent office, the cumulative demand on your focus and patience is real.

Many orthodontists describe it as "quiet exhaustion." They make it through the day without major conflict, but they get home feeling emotionally spent and mentally foggy. Over time, that grind wears down enthusiasm and clouds judgment.

What sets resilient orthodontists apart is not superhuman energy. It is a set of habits and mindsets that help them recover faster and stay present longer.

Three Keys to Staying Sharp:

1. **Protect Your Energy.** Not every question deserves your immediate attention. Not every problem needs to be solved by you. Build a culture where your team handles what they can without you. And don't feel guilty about taking 2–3 quiet moments between patients to reset.

2. **Be Where You Are.** Studies show that "mind-wandering"—thinking about one thing while doing another—correlates directly with unhappiness and fatigue. In other words, worrying about tonight's dinner while placing brackets, or thinking about lab work while answering a parent, drains you faster than the work itself.

   Instead, commit to being fully present in each interaction. You'll feel less scattered and more satisfied at the end of the day.

3. **Recover On Purpose.** You don't recover by default—you recover by design. That means blocking time to move your body, calm your mind, and do something unrelated to orthodontics. Whether it's a workout, a walk, a sauna session, or reading something just for you, build it into your daily and weekly rhythm.

   Even in a low-drama practice, the weight of constant output can take a toll. Mental resilience is about creating systems—internally and externally—that let you show up at your best without burning yourself out in the process.

When you feel better, you lead better. And that's a win for you, your team, and your patients.

The Energy Equation

Energy management—not time management—is the real lever for sustainable performance in your practice. You can't create more hours in a day, but you can absolutely control how much of yourself shows up in each of those hours. And for orthodontists, who balance clinical precision, team dynamics, and high-emotion patient interactions, energy management is non-negotiable.

Think of your capacity like a battery with four distinct cells: **physical, mental, emotional, and purpose-driven energy.** Each drains differently, and each charges differently. Physical energy comes from nutrition, movement, and sleep. Mental energy comes from focus and deliberate breaks. Emotional energy comes from healthy boundaries and positive relationships. And purpose-driven energy comes from staying connected to why you chose this profession in the first place.

THE ENERGY EQUATION

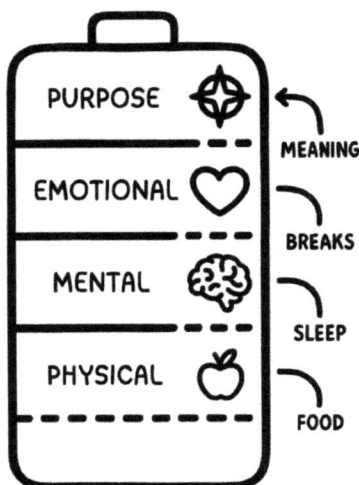

Most clinicians burn through their day reacting, never pausing to see which "cell" is running empty. That's why you feel fine in the morning but drained by mid-afternoon—or why you can't leave work at work when you get home.

Track Your Rhythms

Start by tracking your own patterns. When are you sharpest? Most orthodontists find their cognitive peak in the morning— ideal for treatment planning and high-stakes consultations. Reserve repetitive tasks and lower-stakes cases for the afternoon, when energy naturally dips.

Nutrition is Your Baseline

The brain eats up 20% of your body's total energy, and you can feel it when blood sugar drops: sloppy chairside communication, impatience with a mom's questions, missed details in records. Real food—proteins, vegetables, complex carbs—beats vending-machine fuel every time. A quick mid-morning snack or protein shake can keep your mental edge steady.

Sleep is Your Hidden Multiplier

Poor sleep dulls fine motor control, clouds judgment, and shortens your temper—none of which your patients or team deserve. Good sleep hygiene pays dividends: set a bedtime, keep screens out of the bedroom, and stick to a wind-down routine.

Don't Overlook Emotional and Purpose-Driven Energy

Emotional reserves drain fast when you're managing team conflict or difficult families. Build in ways to recharge: quick walks between patients, music in the office, or even just 5 quiet minutes to reset. Purpose-driven energy gets restored when you reconnect to why you do this—read a thank-you note from a parent, celebrate a team win, or look at the before-and-after photos that remind you why this work matters.

The lesson is simple: **you can't pour from an empty cup.** Managing your energy—on all four levels—is how you show up fully, stay sharp, and make this career sustainable.

Mindful Practice Integration

Mindfulness is all about showing up fully for the moment you're in. That skill is invaluable in an orthodontic or dental practice, where pressure, pace, and people can pull your attention in a dozen directions.

The key is integrating mindfulness into your day, without creating the feeling that you're just adding another thing to your to-do list.

Look for natural transitions such as walking from your office to the operatory, washing your hands, or putting on gloves. These are perfect moments to reset. One deep breath. One mental check-in. One second to quiet your mind and bring your focus back to the patient you are about to see.

You can also anchor mindfulness to routine clinical cues. The sound of sterilization, adjusting your loupes, even hearing your name over the intercom can all remind you to pause and be present. These small rituals keep you grounded even when the day gets chaotic.

Why does it matter? Because patients notice. When you're fully present, they trust you more. You catch subtle signs such as a nervous grip on the chair, hesitation before answering, or confusion. They did not voice that you would miss if you were distracted.

And your team feels it too. **A steady leader brings a steady team.**

The reality of dental and orthodontic practice is that chaos will happen: the schedule will get behind, a patient will show up late, a parent will get demanding. Mindfulness is meant to help you respond to stress instead of reacting to it—keeping your focus where it belongs.

Start small:

- One breath before greeting each patient
- One pause before responding to conflict
- One quiet moment between appointments to reset

These little moments add up. They make you calmer, sharper, and more effective—for your patients, your team, and your-self.

In a high-stakes, high-touch profession, mindfulness is one of the simplest ways to elevate your care and enjoy your work more while you do it.

The Practitioner's Performance Zone

Your clinical results stem not only from your hands, but also from the state of your mind and body.

The best dentists and orthodontists know when they are in the zone. You are fully locked in, focused, steady, and confident. Every movement feels natural. Every decision feels clear. Psychologists call this state "flow," and it is the hallmark of elite performance.

But here's the key: you can't hit flow if your body and mind aren't ready.

Research shows that clinicians who keep their physical health in check—stable blood sugar, regular exercise, proper recovery—access flow nearly four times more often than their burned-out peers. That translates to fewer errors, higher treatment acceptance, and longer careers.

You already train your hands. You need to train your system too.

Why? Because dentistry and orthodontics demand a unique kind of resilience:

- **Precision and posture** - Holding steady, awkward positions for hours while maintaining millimeter-level accuracy, day after day

- **Emotional composure** - Managing anxious or combative patients, high-maintenance parents, and a team that looks to you for calm leadership no matter what

- **Mental clarity under pressure** - Juggling clinical decisions, staff dynamics, and business responsibilities—often all at the same time

- **Relentless schedule demands** - Staying sharp through a packed column of back-to-back patients, with little time to recover between encounters

That combination of stressors requires systems built specifically for this profession—like chairside ergonomics to save your neck and back, movement or breathing resets between patients, and nutrition habits that keep you sharp through a full schedule.

Even your practice environment impacts your performance zone. Poor lighting, noisy hallways, awkward operatory setups—all sap your energy and make precision harder. The smartest clinicians treat their environment as part of their toolkit, not an afterthought. A well-designed operatory helps you stay in flow longer, perform more procedures with less strain, and leave work feeling less depleted.

Here's the takeaway: Your skillset is only as good as the state you bring to the chair. Every improvement you make to your physical readiness, mental sharpness, and practice environment is a clinical performance upgrade.

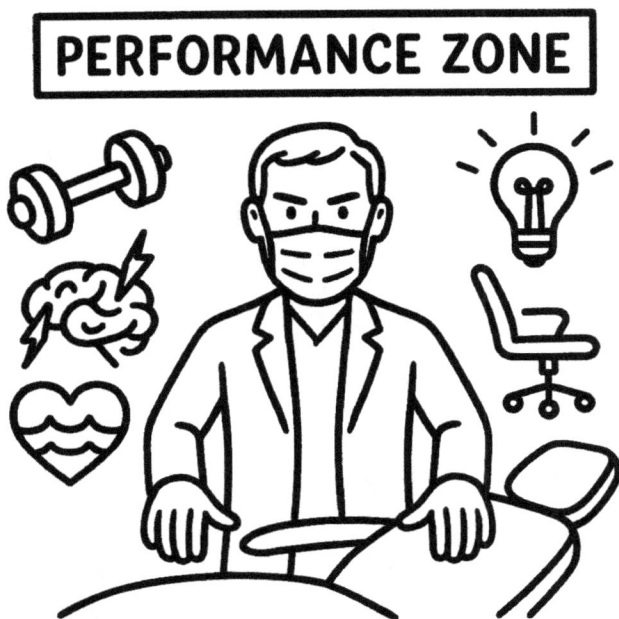

If you want to stay at your best for your patients, your team, and yourself, build and protect your performance zone as if it were your most valuable asset. Because it is.

The Resilience Protocol

Resilience comes from creating systems you can actually sustain, not from grinding harder.

The best clinicians treat their own wellbeing the same way they approach orthodontics—with a plan, measured progress, and consistent habits.

Habit Stacking

One proven tactic is habit stacking: attach a beneficial action to something you already do.

- After every bonding or adjustment, take 60 seconds to stretch your neck and shoulders before moving to the next chair
- When sanitizing and gloving up, take three slow breaths to reset before seeing the next patient

Consistency Beats Intensity

Fifteen minutes of exercise you actually stick to is better than sporadic, punishing sessions. Likewise, three minutes of mindfulness between patients is better than a 30-minute practice you never do.

Find your minimum effective dose—the smallest routine that delivers the biggest return—and make it non-negotiable.

Track What Matters

Vague goals like "stress less" don't work. Measure the things that directly affect how you perform:

- **Resting heart rate variability (HRV)** - a key marker of resilience and recovery

- **Sleep quality** - which fuels mental clarity and emotional control
- **Movement goals** - so your body doesn't break down from static posture

Wearables like WHOOP, Oura, or Garmin are worth the investment. They give you hard data about how your body is responding—showing you trends in recovery, sleep, and strain that you'd otherwise miss. When you can see the numbers, you're more likely to adjust your habits and stay on track.

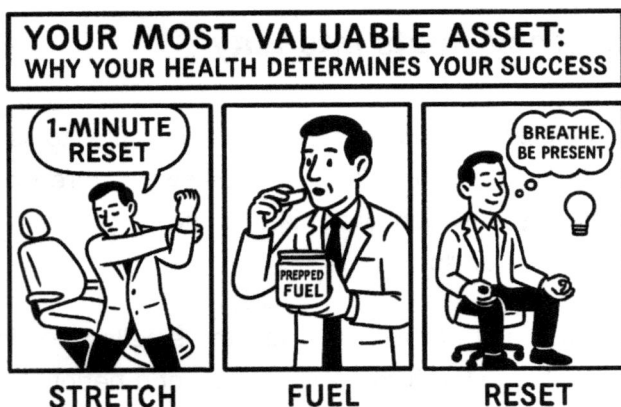

YOUR MOST VALUABLE ASSET:
WHY YOUR HEALTH DETERMINES YOUR SUCCESS

STRETCH   FUEL   RESET

Plan for the Hard Weeks

Busy seasons will happen, so be ready to adapt with them.

- A no-excuses, 10-minute bodyweight workout you can do in your office
- Prepped healthy snacks so you're not grabbing candy from the drawer

- A short mindfulness reset you can use in between back-to-back patients

Recovery is Part of Training

Recovery keeps you in the game longer:

- Contrast therapy (hot and cold) to reduce inflammation
- Compression boots or sleeves to restore circulation
- Trigger point release and targeted massage to undo the strain of clinical work

The real question is: How much better could you perform—for your patients, your team, and your family—if you stopped just "pushing through" and started showing up at your best, every day?

Implementing Your Wellbeing Protocol

Your health habits need a solid system. The same principles you use to run a smooth practice also apply here: assess, prioritize, and simplify.

Start by taking stock: Where do you feel drained? Sleep, movement, stress, focus? Then pick one small, high-impact change. Add protein to every meal before worrying about perfect nutrition. Take 5 minutes to stretch between patients before signing up for a marathon. Early wins build momentum.

Set up your environment for success. Lay out gym clothes the night before. Keep healthy snacks where you'd normally reach for candy. Use phone reminders or apps to block time for breaks and track progress. The less you rely on willpower, the more consistent you'll be.

Accountability helps. Some clinicians buddy up with a peer, others use apps, and many bring their team into the mix. A shared wellness challenge in your office benefits everyone—and keeps you honest.

Most importantly, stop framing health as separate from your professional life. Your habits are not optional extras. They form the foundation that supports the level of care and leadership you strive to deliver. When you see wellbeing as part of your professional identity, consistency comes naturally.

The Vital Connection Between Health and Practice Success

Your health is your greatest professional asset. When you neglect it, the effects show up in your work, your team, and your patients.

Sustainable health routines don't require drastic change. The secret is consistency: small actions that build resilience and keep you steady through the inevitable storms of running a practice.

Mindfulness is one of the most powerful tools in your kit. It goes beyond stress relief and directly improves how you show up as a leader and clinician. Dentists who practice mindfulness make clearer decisions, communicate better with patients and staff, and resist the urge to micromanage their team.

This is the real value of delegation: when you're healthy and balanced, you're better at letting go of what doesn't need your direct attention. The time and headspace you reclaim become fuel for the routines that keep you at your best.

Don't fall into the trap of thinking self-care is selfish. It's how you make your practice, your relationships, and your career sustainable. Your team needs a leader who's clear-eyed and fully engaged. Your family needs you to come home whole. And you deserve to enjoy the life you've built.

You can keep sacrificing your health for short-term productivity—or you can choose the smarter path: investing in yourself to unlock your full potential at work and beyond.

The choice is yours. Make it count.

Luke's Biohacking & Health Recommendations

I've spent years experimenting with what actually works—not just what sounds good on a podcast. Here are the tools, protocols, and tests I personally use and recommend.

Sleep Like a Billionaire

Tom Ferriss, who has interviewed some of the world's most successful people, says their number one hack is sleeping on a cold surface. And it works. Your body recovers better and sleeps deeper in a cooler environment. Studies show optimal sleep happens between 60–67°F.

I use: Perfectly Snug

Cold Plunging: The Legal Drug

Nothing wakes me up, clears my head, and lowers inflammation faster than a cold plunge. It boosts energy, improves mood, and strengthens your immune system.

I use: The Plunge tub at home and their portable unit when I travel.

Track What Matters

I've worn a Whoop for six years. It gives you actionable insights on how sleep, travel, alcohol, and stress really affect you. Eye-opening.

I use: Whoop

Red Light Therapy

If you can't get early morning sun, red light therapy is the next best thing. It improves circadian rhythm, energy, and recovery.

I use: TheraLight Bed, but you can start with something much more affordable.

Sweat Like You're Supposed To

Your body was made to sweat. Saunas have proven cardiovascular and detox benefits. Frequent sauna use is linked to significantly lower mortality rates.

I use: Sunlighten infrared sauna.

Biomat: Recover and Relax

I was reminded how effective biomats are when a friend borrowed mine for a back injury. Great for pain, stress, and circulation.

I use: Biomat

The Biohacker's Bath

My go-to when I feel rundown or inflamed:

- Water that's as hot as you can stand
- 2 cups Epsom salt
- 1/2 cup baking soda
- 1/2 cup food-grade hydrogen peroxide

Sit for 20 minutes.

Fix Your Diet

If you can't lose weight, try a strict Autoimmune Paleo (AIP) diet. No cheats. Zero. If you haven't dropped weight in 90 days on AIP, I'd be shocked.

Run the Right Labs

If you feel off and your doctor "can't find anything," get serious testing:

- Stool test (gut health)
- Mineral test
- Autoimmune panel
- Full thyroid panel
- Full hormone panel
- Lyme test if symptoms fit

Mainstream doctors miss this stuff all the time—and it's a huge contributor to today's chronic illness epidemic.

If you want to talk health, wellness, or need help getting started, email me directly: Luke@hipcreativeinc.com

Your health is your foundation. Protect it, improve it, and watch everything else improve with it.

Key Takeaways

- Your health is the foundation of your practice. Neglecting it harms you, your patients, and your team.
- Energy management (physical, mental, emotional, purpose-driven) is more critical than time management.
- Mindfulness and presence directly improve leadership, communication, and patient trust.
- Recovery and resilience protocols are non-negotiable for long-term sustainability.
- Delegation and systems free up time for self-care, creating a virtuous cycle of health and success.

Next Steps

You don't need to overhaul your entire lifestyle to reclaim your health. Starting this week, you can:

Identify one health habit to improve—nutrition, sleep, movement, or recovery—and make it consistent.

Block non-negotiable recovery time into your schedule— whether that's a workout, a walk, or a mindfulness practice.

Share one wellbeing goal with your team or family for accountability and support.

Taking care of your health is the foundation of everything. Without energy, clarity, and resilience, no system, team, or practice model can sustain you. But once your most valuable asset is protected and running at its best, the next step is to think beyond yourself.

That's where wealth-building comes in. Your clinical skill and reputation are powerful, but they're finite if every dollar depends on your time in the chair. To create lasting freedom, you need assets that work for you while you sleep. In the next chapter, we'll explore how entrepreneurial opportunities and passive income can transform your financial future so that the practice you've built doesn't just sustain your health and lifestyle, but also funds the life you truly want to live.

Chapter 11: Entrepreneurial Opportunities and Passive Income

By: Luke Infinger

Dr. Steve sat across from his old residency buddy at their favorite steakhouse, the same place they had celebrated matching into their programs fifteen years ago. But tonight, Steve wasn't celebrating. He was exhausted—still trading hours for dollars, grinding chairside every day, and feeling like the life he had built was slowly owning him instead of the other way around.

Across the table, Bob was buzzing with energy, talking about investments that worked for him while he slept. Steve forced a smile, but inside, he felt the gut punch. Somewhere along the way, Bob had built wealth. Steve had only built a job.

The path to long-term freedom as a dentist or orthodontist isn't found in working more hours or squeezing in more patients. True wealth and true sustainability come from diversification. By expanding beyond chairside production into entrepreneurial opportunities and passive income streams, you transform your practice from your only asset into the foundation for multiple revenue streams. Done right, this shift allows you to reclaim your time, protect your health, and build lasting wealth that supports both your practice and your life.

In this chapter, you'll learn why relying solely on clinical income caps your potential, how to identify entrepreneurial opportunities that align with your practice persona, and what passive income streams can work for you. Most importantly, you'll see how to diversify without distraction so your core practice thrives while your wealth multiplies in the background.

Beyond the Chair: Are You Missing Life-Changing Revenue Streams?

The True Cost of Singular Focus

Your practice holds more potential than you realize. While most clinicians focus exclusively on direct patient care, a select few have discovered that clinical excellence is just the beginning. The traditional model—work more hours, see more patients, make more money—leads straight to burnout for many talented clinicians. This exhausting cycle represents what I call the Practice Paradox: the very system designed to reward your expertise simultaneously threatens your wellbeing and longevity in the profession.

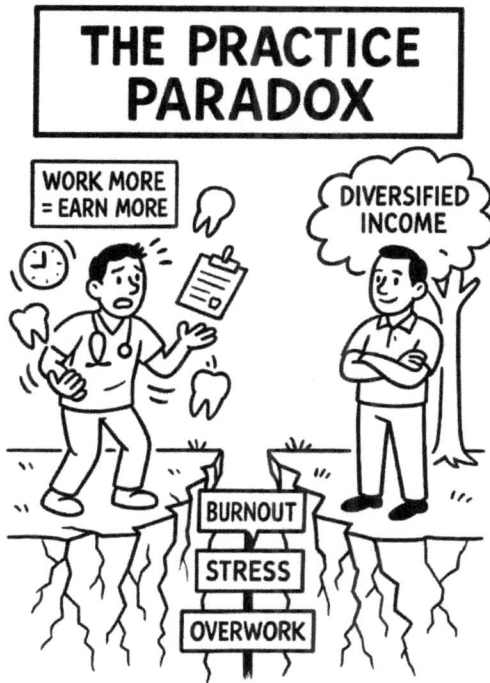

The most successful clinicians understand something fundamental: **sustainability requires diversification.** Think about it—you've invested years mastering complex clinical skills and building patient trust. This intellectual and relationship capital creates opportunities that extend far beyond traditional chairside revenue. Yet most healthcare professionals never leverage these assets fully, leaving significant potential unrealized while working themselves to exhaustion.

What separates thriving, balanced practices from those where owners feel trapped? The answer lies in understanding your unique practice persona. Not every dentist or orthodontist wants the same things or functions optimally under identical conditions. Some thrive as clinical perfectionists, others as business strategists, and still others as lifestyle clinicians. **Recognizing your authentic professional identity is the critical first step toward building a practice model that generates both wealth and wellbeing.**

The Entrepreneurial Mindset Shift

The entrepreneurial clinician sees beyond conventional boundaries. While maintaining clinical excellence, they recognize their expertise can be monetized through multiple channels that complement rather than compete with patient care. This perspective shift doesn't require abandoning your clinical identity—quite the opposite. It means leveraging that identity to create value in ways that don't demand your constant physical presence.

Consider the stark reality: there's a ceiling to what you can earn through direct patient care alone. Even at maximum efficiency, there are only so many hours in a day and procedures you can perform. **The path to true financial freedom requires building systems that generate revenue while you sleep.** This isn't about cutting corners clinically—it's about expanding your impact while reclaiming your time.

The most fulfilling practices emerge when you align your business model with your core values and strengths. Some clinicians find joy in creating educational content that helps colleagues improve their skills. Others develop products that solve common clinical challenges. Still others invest in real estate or build referral networks that create mutual benefit. The key is identifying opportunities that energize rather than deplete you.

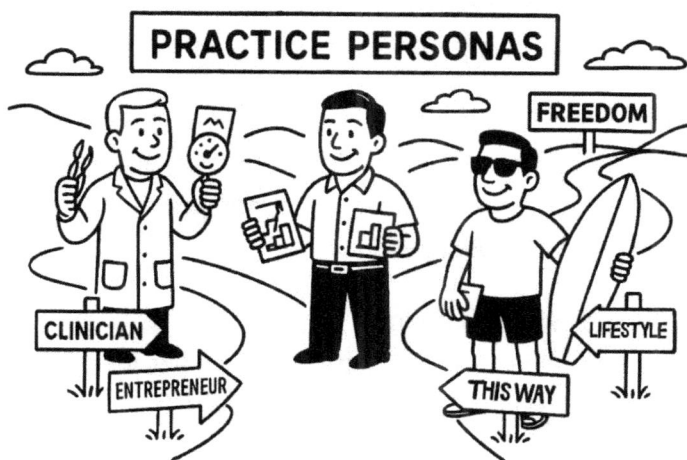

The Wake-Up Call

The details spilled out over dinner. Bob had bought into a surgery center, partnered on a medical spa, and built equity in the building where his practice was located, collecting rent from other specialists every month. He even created a captive insurance company that not only reduced his taxes but also grew wealth he could pass on to his kids.

When Steve finally asked how much of Bob's income came from outside the chair, Bob didn't hesitate.

"About sixty percent," he said. "And I spend maybe two hours a month managing it."

Steve's stomach sank. He thought about his own situation: leasing a building that was making his landlord rich, working sixty hours a week, relying entirely on a practice that would stop paying him the second he stopped working.

Driving home that night, Steve couldn't shake the conversation. For the first time, he saw the truth: the ceiling on his income wasn't his skill; it was his mindset. If he wanted real freedom, he couldn't just work harder; he had to think differently.

Beyond Clinical Practice: Strategic Revenue Expansion

For Orthodontists: Master Your Core First

Here's the hard truth most orthodontists don't want to hear: stop looking for other opportunities and dial in orthodontics. It's almost more profitable than anything else you could pursue.

The margins are exceptional, the demand is consistent, and you've already invested years mastering the skills.

Before chasing external revenue streams, maximize what you already have:

- **Optimize case flow** - Streamline patient scheduling and treatment protocols
- **Improve case acceptance** - What percentage of consultations start treatment?
- **Expand and/or improve treatment options** - Whitening, Retainer Plans, Aligners with better quality/lower lab fee, esthetics
- **Perfect your systems** - Reduce no-shows, maximize chair time, eliminate bottlenecks

But there are strategic additions that make sense:

Aesthetics Integration Injectables represent one of the easiest practice add-ons with exceptional margins. Injectables and dermal fillers complement orthodontic treatment perfectly—patients who invest in straight teeth often want comprehensive facial aesthetics. The training is straightforward, the ROI is immediate, and it positions you as a complete smile transformation provider.

Strategic Staffing Solutions Most orthodontists avoid hiring general dentists because they fear upsetting referring doctors. But consider this game-changing approach: **What if you had a dentist on staff for dental clearance?**

Benefits:

- Handle debonds with high-speed drills (faster than orthodontists)
- Eliminate dental clearance bottlenecks that slow treatment
- Generate additional revenue through basic restorative work
- Provide convenience that patients love

Even bolder: Add an oral surgeon. Most kids need wisdom teeth removed after finishing treatment. Instead of referring out, you capture that revenue and provide one-stop convenience for families.

For General Dentists: Leverage Your Foundation

General dentistry offers more diversification opportunities than any other dental specialty:

High-Margin Add-Ons

- **Cosmetic procedures** - Veneers, whitening, smile makeovers
- **Implant placement** - Both surgical and restorative phases

- **Sleep medicine** - Oral appliances for sleep apnea (huge untapped market)
- Injectables - Fillers with dental-specific training

Ancillary Revenue Streams

- **In-house lab work** - Crown and bridge, night guards, appliances
- **Hygiene expansion** - Additional hygienists, extended hours
- **Specialty services** - Endodontics, periodontics, oral surgery

Real Estate: Your Practice Foundation

The Single Most Important Decision: Do You Own Your Building?

Owning your practice real estate creates multiple benefits:

- **Equity building** - Convert monthly rent expense into long-term investment
- **Control** - No landlord dictating lease terms or practice environment
- **Tax advantages** - Depreciation, interest deductions, business expense benefits

- **Rental income** - Lease space to compatible healthcare providers
- **Retirement asset** - Sell building separate from practice for maximum value

The numbers are compelling: Instead of paying $8,000/month rent ($96,000/year) for 20 years ($1.92 million), you could own an appreciating asset worth $2-3 million.

Satellite Location Strategy

If you have satellite locations you visit only a few days monthly:

- **Sublease to specialists** on your off days (oral surgeons, periodontists)
- **Shared space agreements** with complementary providers
- **Equipment partnerships** - Let colleagues use your technology for fee splits

Real Estate Investment Beyond Your Practice

- **Medical office buildings** - Leverage your healthcare market knowledge
- **Dental practice real estate** - Buy buildings and lease to colleagues
- **Residential rental properties** - Traditional passive income

- **Real estate investment trusts (REITs)** - Professional management, diversification

Adjacent Business Opportunities: Leveraging Your Local Influence

Your professional credibility and local network create investment opportunities others can't access:

Healthcare-Adjacent Businesses

- **Med spas** - Partner as investor and board member
- **Chiropractic practices** - Cross-referral opportunities, shared patient base
- **Surgery centers** - Ambulatory surgical centers serving your market (or similar)
- **Urgent care centers** - Capture overflow from medical practices

Investment Partnerships. Use your local influence to be brought in as an investor and board member:

- **Professional service businesses** - Accounting, legal, consulting firms serving healthcare
- **Healthcare startups** - Angel investing in dental/medical technology
- **Local business ventures** - Leverage your professional reputation

Personal Financial Architecture: Building Real Wealth

The Flow System

The saddest conversations I have are with high-income earners who are broke. Orthodontists making $500,000+ annually but living paycheck to paycheck. **You must fix this immediately.**

Organize your finances like a business with clear systems:

Main Account (Revenue Hub) All practice and investment income flows here first.

Monthly Distributions:

- **Bills Account (Fixed Costs)** - Mortgage, utilities, insurance, loan payments
- **Spend Account (Lifestyle)** - You and spouse's discretionary money with limits
- **Investment Account (Wealth Building)** - 10-30% minimum, non-negotiable
- **Emergency Fund** - 6-12 months expenses, separate high-yield account

Strategic Wealth Building

Money Doubling: The Rule of 72 Money doubles every 7.2 years at 10% return. A 35-year-old investing $100,000 will have $800,000 at age 65. **Time is your most valuable asset.**

Dollar-Cost Averaging Bitcoin Data shows consistent Bitcoin purchasing beats timing the market. Consider 1-5% of portfolio allocation for long-term wealth preservation. Personally, I (Luke) started investing in Bitcoin in 2018, buying small amounts twice a month. I am now up 74% and kicking myself for not investing more. In my opinion, Bitcoin is now mainstream and even our current administration is bullish on crypto. I would not recommend investing in 99% of coins unless you do your research. Most outside Bitcoin will never amount to anything.

Hedging Against Dollar Devaluation

- **Luxury collectibles** - Rolex watches, rare handbags, collector cars (things that hold value and you can enjoy)
- **Precious metals** - Gold and silver for portfolio insurance
- **Real assets** - Land, buildings, tangible investments

Avoid Depreciating "Assets" Boats are money pits. Water ruins everything. If it doesn't appreciate or generate income, think twice. Focus on assets that work for you.

Advanced Tax and Wealth Strategies

Whole Life Insurance and Infinite Banking

For younger practitioners (under 45), whole life insurance offers unique benefits:

- **Tax-free growth** - Cash value accumulates without current taxation
- **Tax-free loans** - Borrow against cash value for investments or major purchases
- **Estate planning** - Death benefit provides family protection
- **Infinite banking concept** - Use policy as personal bank, pay yourself interest

Captive Insurance Companies

For high-net-worth orthodontists and dentists ($1M+ annual income):

- **Self-insurance** - Cover practice risks internally instead of paying insurance companies
- **Tax deductions** - Premium payments reduce taxable income significantly

- **Investment growth** - Captive assets grow tax-deferred
- **Family wealth transfer** - Pass captive ownership to children for generational wealth

Estate Planning Essentials

Will and Testament Without a will, state intestacy laws determine who gets your assets. Probate can consume 5-10% of estate value and take years. This is malpractice for high-income professionals.

Trust Structures

- **Revocable living trusts** - Avoid probate, maintain control during lifetime
- **Irrevocable life insurance trusts** - Remove life insurance from taxable estate
- **Generation-skipping trusts** - Benefit grandchildren directly, skip estate taxes

Are You Actually Creating Wealth?

The harsh reality check: Are you building wealth or just earning a high income?

Wealth Building Indicators:

- **Net worth grows faster than income** - Assets appreciating beyond salary
- **Passive income streams** - Money earned without trading time
- **Investment portfolio** - Diversified holdings beyond practice equity
- **Multiple revenue sources** - Not dependent on chair time alone

High-Income, Zero-Wealth Red Flags:

- Living paycheck to paycheck despite high earnings
- No emergency fund or investment accounts
- All wealth tied up in practice equity
- Lifestyle inflation matches income increases

Always live BELOW your means. The goal isn't to spend what you make—it's to invest what you don't spend.

Passive Income: The Healthcare Professional's Path to Freedom

Passive income represents the holy grail for healthcare professionals—earning money while you sleep, vacation, or focus on the clinical work you love most. Unlike direct patient care, which requires your physical presence and active time investment, passive income continues flowing with minimal ongoing effort after initial setup.

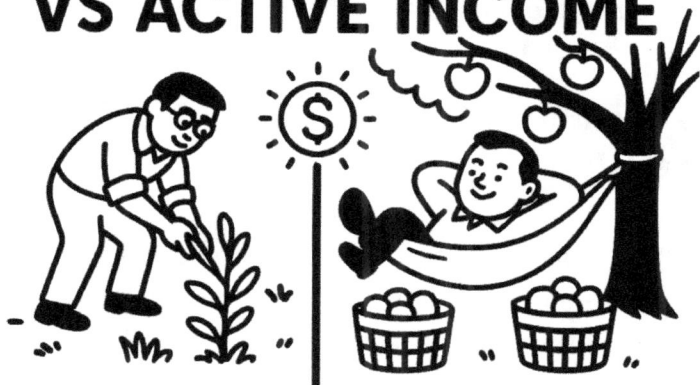

Picture passive income as planting fruit trees rather than growing annual vegetables. The initial investment of time, money, and effort is substantial—selecting the right varieties, preparing the soil, and nurturing young saplings. But once established, these trees produce fruit year after year with only periodic maintenance, while vegetables must be replanted each season, requiring constant attention and work.

Examples of healthcare professional passive income:

- **Real estate investments** - Medical office buildings, rental properties
- **Royalties** - Books, educational products, course materials

- **Intellectual property** - Patented devices, treatment protocols
- **Investment portfolios** - Stocks, bonds, REITs, index funds
- **Business ownership** - Equity stakes in dental labs, supply companies

The Mental Shift: From Time-for-Money to Assets-for-Money

Most healthcare professionals have been trained to trade time for money—more patients, more procedures, more hours equals more income. Passive income inverts this equation, focusing instead on creating or acquiring assets that work for you.

This mental adjustment can be challenging for clinicians accustomed to direct service delivery, but it's essential for long-term wealth building and practice sustainability.

Finding the Perfect Complement to Your Practice

Selecting entrepreneurial opportunities that enhance rather than detract from your primary practice requires strategic thinking. The ideal complementary ventures leverage your existing resources, align with your practice values, and create synergies rather than competition for your time and energy.

Start by conducting an honest inventory of your practice's underutilized assets:

- **Empty operatories** during certain days or hours
- **Administrative staff** with capacity for additional responsibilities
- **Marketing channels** reaching your patient base
- **Treatment rooms** that could accommodate allied health professionals
- **Technology investments** that could serve other practitioners

Consider your practice like an established oak tree with a strong root system. The wisest approach isn't planting competing trees that fight for the same sunlight and nutrients, but rather adding complementary plants that thrive in the environment you've already created.

Strategic partnerships often provide the best complementary revenue opportunities:

- **Specialist arrangements** - In-house procedures, space-sharing
- **Compatible healthcare providers** - Physical therapy, nutrition counseling
- **Technology sharing** - Digital scanners, 3D printing, milling equipment

Remember: complementary opportunities should align with your practice personality types and professional goals. The most sustainable additions will feel energizing rather than draining, creating professional satisfaction alongside financial returns.

The Revenue Diversification Framework

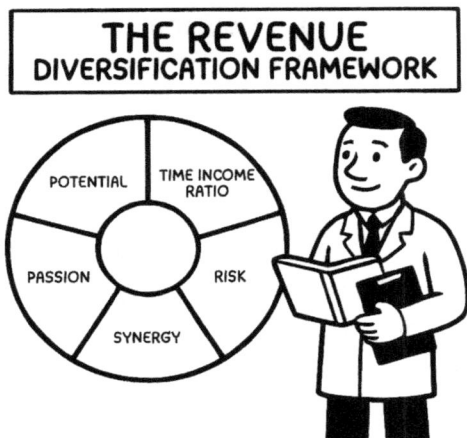

THE REVENUE DIVERSIFICATION FRAMEWORK

POTENTIAL | TIME INCOME RATIO | PASSION | RISK | SYNERGY

Before pursuing additional income streams, establish clear criteria for evaluation:

Five Evaluation Factors:

1. **Synergy with existing practice** - Does it leverage current infrastructure, team, or patient base?

2. **Passion alignment** - Will you find it intellectually stimulating and personally satisfying?

3. **Time-to-income ratio** - How much effort is required relative to potential returns?

4. **Long-term potential** - Can it grow into significant income or remain complementary?

5. **Risk profile** - What financial, reputational, or regulatory risks does it present?

This framework helps filter opportunities through both business and personal lenses, ensuring you pursue ventures aligned with your overall goals.

A Tale of Two Dentists: Contrasting Approaches

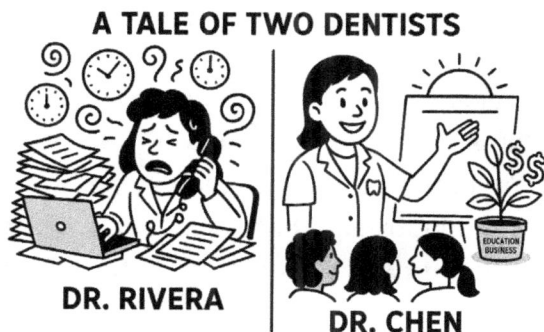

A TALE OF TWO DENTISTS

DR. RIVERA

DR. CHEN

Dr. Rivera and Dr. Chen graduated dental school together ten years ago. Both built successful practices, but their approaches to income diversification couldn't be more different.

Dr. Rivera, driven by desire for immediate income, jumped at every opportunity—investing in a dental product startup, purchasing rental properties, starting a consulting business, and developing patient education software. With attention divided between numerous ventures, her core practice suffered. Team members complained about her absence, patients noted declining service quality, and she worked constantly yet felt perpetually behind.

Dr. Chen took a methodical approach. She first maximized her practice efficiency, then carefully evaluated complementary opportunities against her strengths and interests. Recognizing her teaching abilities and underutilized operatories on Fridays, she developed a hands-on implant course for general dentists. This single focus allowed her to build a respected continuing education program that generated substantial passive income while enhancing her clinical reputation.

Ten years later, Dr. Rivera has abandoned most ventures after minimal returns, while Dr. Chen earns 40% of her income from her education business with just one day per week invested. **The contrast illustrates that successful diversification isn't about quantity of ventures but strategic alignment with your strengths, resources, and goals.**

The Ultimate Practice Freedom

"Financial independence gives you the freedom to focus on excellence rather than volume. When you're not dependent solely on direct patient care for income, you can make practice decisions based on quality and satisfaction rather than necessity." - Dr. Howard Farran, founder of Dentaltown

When financial pressure diminishes, you can:

- Spend more time with complex patients
- Create space for family priorities and personal health
- Invest in advanced education without immediate ROI pressure
- Take more vacations without income anxiety
- Transition gradually toward retirement

This freedom represents the ultimate practice paradox resolution—building business success that enhances rather than sacrifices personal wellbeing.

Beyond the Chair: Expanding Your Professional Horizons

Building entrepreneurial opportunities and passive income streams isn't just about making more money—it's about creating sustainability in your practice and your life. The strategies we've explored offer pathways to reduce your dependence on chair time while maximizing your professional impact and personal freedom.

Your expertise as a healthcare professional is valuable beyond direct patient care. By diversifying your revenue streams through real estate, strategic investments, and complementary business ventures, you transform knowledge that took years to acquire into assets that work for you even when you aren't.

The practice paradox reveals itself clearly in this domain: by thoughtfully expanding beyond traditional practice boundaries, you can actually create more freedom within them. Healthcare professionals who develop multiple income streams often find they practice with greater joy and intention when patient care becomes a choice rather than their sole financial lifeline.

Perhaps most importantly, the entrepreneurial ventures you choose must align with your practice persona and core values. The right opportunities will complement rather than compete with your primary practice, creating synergy instead of strain.

Your journey toward practice fulfillment isn't limited to clinical excellence alone. By embracing the entrepreneurial opportunities that resonate with your unique practice persona, you create a professional life that reflects your true aspirations—one where burnout fades and balance becomes not just possible, but inevitable.

The path forward is yours to design. Start small, stay aligned with your values, and remember that the ultimate goal isn't maximizing income—it's maximizing fulfillment while maintaining the freedom to practice on your own terms.

Most importantly: Are you actually creating wealth, or are you just a high-income earner living paycheck to paycheck? Fix this first—everything else is just details.

Important Disclaimer

The information provided in this chapter is for educational and informational purposes only and should not be construed as financial, investment, tax, or legal advice.

The authors are not licensed financial advisors, investment professionals, tax advisors, or attorneys. All strategies, examples, and recommendations discussed are based on personal opinion and general industry observations. Every individual's financial situation is unique, and what works for one person may not be appropriate for another.

Before making any financial, investment, or business decisions:

- Consult with qualified professionals including financial advisors, tax professionals, attorneys, and accountants
- Conduct your own due diligence and research
- Consider your personal risk tolerance and financial circumstances
- Understand that all investments carry risk and potential for loss

The authors assume no responsibility or liability for any decisions made by readers based on the information presented in this chapter. Past performance does not guarantee future results. Market conditions, tax laws, and regulations can change and may affect the suitability of any strategy discussed.

Readers are encouraged to seek professional guidance tailored to their specific circumstances before implementing any financial, investment, or business strategy mentioned in this material.

Key Takeaways

- Chairside income alone caps your freedom. Diversification is essential.

- Your reputation, patient trust, and professional network are underutilized assets.

- Passive income streams (real estate, partnerships, IP, investments) build wealth without demanding constant presence.

- Align entrepreneurial opportunities with your practice persona and values to avoid burnout.

- True financial freedom is not about maximizing income; it's about maximizing your life. It's about maximizing fulfillment while maintaining choice and balance.

Next Steps

You don't need to build everything at once. Start small and strategic:

Evaluate complementary opportunities – Look at med spas, CE courses, or products that align with your practice.

Protect your wealth – Explore trusts, insurance structures, and tax strategies with the guidance of professionals.

Set a diversification goal – Aim to generate at least 20–30% of your income outside the chair within 5–10 years.

Creating assets and building streams of passive income unlocks new levels of freedom. You no longer rely solely on chairside hours to provide for your family or fund your future. However, the most successful practitioners know that freedom without direction quickly turns into distraction. The deeper question is: **What are you building it all for?**

This is where purpose comes into play. Without a clearly defined sense of "enough" and a calling that gives meaning to your work, even the smartest investments and entrepreneurial wins can leave you feeling empty. In the next chapter, we'll explore how to align your practice, wealth, and systems with the higher purpose of your life, so that everything you do contributes not just to income, but also to impact and legacy.

Section VI: Purpose & Reflection

Discover:

Chapter 12 – What's the Purpose of Life and Your Practice?: How defining "enough" and aligning your work with your higher purpose creates meaning beyond metrics.

Chapter 13 – Your Next Steps: How to turn insight into action with a clear framework for implementation, ensuring your practice serves your life rather than consuming it.

Chapter 12: What's the Purpose of Life and Your Practice?

By: Dr. Kyle Fagala

Dr. Antonio had every marker of success a clinician could dream of—multiple thriving locations, steady year-over-year growth, associates carrying the load, and his name respected in the community. Yet at forty-five, staring at another glowing quarterly report, he felt a deep, unsettling emptiness. The more he built, the more it seemed to cost him. Family dinners were missed. Kids' games were unattended. His wife stopped asking when he'd be home. Externally, everything looked perfect. Internally, it wasn't enough. No number on a balance sheet could fill the hollow space where meaning was supposed to live.

This is the paradox at the heart of this chapter: chasing "more" without defining what *enough* means will leave you burned out, disconnected, and empty. True success isn't measured by production, locations, or external accolades. It's measured by alignment between your practice and your deeper purpose in life. When you build systems that serve not just your business but your calling, you create space for joy, presence, and legacy that no amount of "more" can buy.

This chapter asks the deeper question: *What is all this for?* What's the purpose of your practice and your life? Defining "enough" isn't about settling. It's about reclaiming your time and aligning your practice with your highest values so you can live with intention. Whether your deeper purpose is faith, family, service, or legacy, the ultimate paradox is this: the more effectively you build systems that free you from busyness, the more you're able to invest in the things that actually matter.

Why "Enough" Might Be the Most Powerful Word in Your Professional Vocabulary

Here's the truth they don't teach you in dental school: **time is the only currency that actually matters.**

You can make more money. You can see more patients. You can open more locations. But you can't make more time. Every hour you spend trapped in your practice, micromanaging details that someone else could handle, is an hour stolen from your real purpose in life.

And that purpose? It's bigger than perfect occlusion, bigger than five-star Google reviews, bigger than the newest CBCT machine. Your deeper purpose—whether it's glorifying God and serving His creation, raising children who change the world, or whatever calling stirs your soul—can't happen if you're forever chained to operatory schedules and insurance claims.

This is the ultimate practice paradox: the better you become at building systems that work without you, the more freedom you gain to focus on what actually matters.

The Growth Trap That's Stealing Your Life

The relentless pursuit of growth has become the unquestioned dogma of dentistry and orthodontics. We chase bigger patient rosters, expanded service offerings, multiple locations with such certainty that we rarely stop to ask: "Why?"

The truth that many successful orthodontists eventually discover—often after years of exhaustion—is that the growth-at-all-costs mindset creates a treadmill with no off switch.

Success without purpose is simply busy work dressed in expensive scrubs. I've watched countless dentists build impressive practices while simultaneously constructing gilded cages for themselves. They reach their production targets only to discover an emptiness that no balance sheet can fill.

This emptiness demonstrates a deeper discovery: that the most insidious trap in professional practice isn't failure—it's succeeding at the wrong thing.

Many orthodontists measure themselves against industry benchmarks that have no relevance to their actual life goals.

They celebrate doubling their patient base while their personal relationships wither. They expand into multiple locations while their health deteriorates. They achieve clinical recognition while missing their kids' childhood.

The Weight of More

As Dr. Antonio sat in his darkened office, the quarterly reports glowed on the desk in front of him. On paper, his practice was thriving—twenty-three percent growth, new associates on board, and another location in development. But all he could think about was his daughter's question at dinner the week before: *"Dad, when was the last time you actually spent a whole day seeing patients without running off to meetings?"* He hadn't known how to answer.

That question echoed now, louder than the numbers staring back at him. He remembered when orthodontics had been pure joy—the energy of the clinic, the excitement of watching a child's smile transform. But somewhere along the way, the joy had been buried under expansion plans, leadership meetings, and endless spreadsheets. He realized that success had become about chasing "more"—

more patients, more locations, more accolades—while the very purpose of his life and practice slipped away.

It dawned on him that he had never defined what *enough* looked like. Enough income to live well without sacrificing family dinners. Enough patients to feel meaningful impact without drowning in volume. Enough time to be present with the people who mattered most. The reports measured growth, but they couldn't measure what he was losing.

Antonio's story reveals the deeper truth: without a clear definition of *enough,* growth becomes a treadmill. The higher purpose that gives work meaning gets crowded out by endless pursuit. For him, the breakthrough wasn't another layer of expansion but a realignment. A recognition that the numbers only mattered when they served a purpose bigger than themselves.

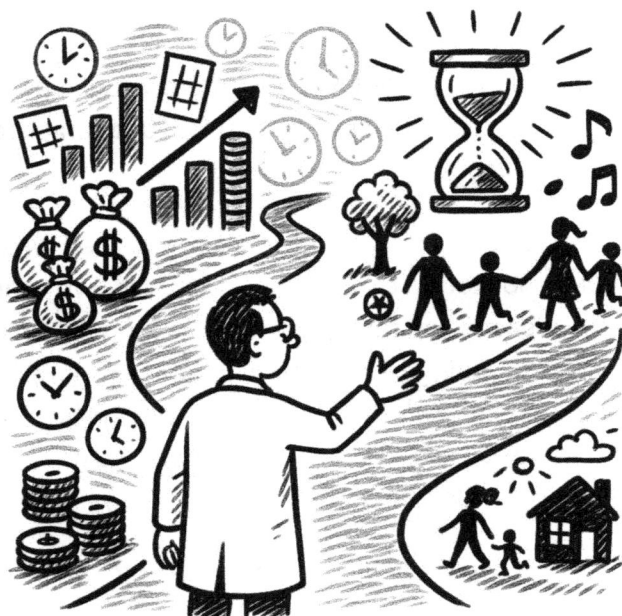

Time: The Ultimate Currency

Time is the ultimate currency because it's the only resource you can't create more of, save for later, borrow against the future, or recover once spent.

Every hour you spend on tasks that could be delegated is an hour stolen from activities only you can do—whether that's complex clinical cases, mentoring young orthodontists, serving your community, or being present with your family.

Consider the mathematics of time investment. If you spend two hours weekly on administrative tasks that a properly trained team member could handle, that's 104 hours per year—more than two full work weeks—of your irreplaceable time being misallocated.

The orthodontists who understand time as the ultimate currency make dramatically different choices about practice structure. They invest heavily in systems that buy back their time, even when the initial cost seems high. They hire and train exceptional team members, recognizing that the upfront investment pays dividends in reclaimed hours for years to come.

Dr. Patricia transformed her practice by applying this time-currency mindset. She realized she was spending fifteen minutes per patient on routine documentation that a well-trained assistant could handle in five minutes. By training her team and implementing digital workflows, she reclaimed nearly ten hours per week—time she now invests in complex clinical cases, continuing education, and family activities that had been neglected for years.

Many orthodontists in similar situations report a shift in perspective: what initially seems like an expense for better systems becomes an investment in reclaiming their most valuable resource. The time saved often proves more valuable than revenue increases alone, allowing practitioners to focus on the clinical work they're passionate about while maintaining a healthier work-life balance.

The Practice Personality Types Revisited: Finding Your "Enough"

Throughout this book, we've explored six distinct practice personality types. When viewed through the lens of purpose and "enough," these personalities reveal different relationships with growth, time, and meaning.

The Tech-Forward Office finds "enough" in perfecting innovative care delivery rather than endlessly scaling. Dr. Jason Yang's focus on CBCT imaging, 3D printing, and advanced procedures represents this approach—constantly improving the quality and efficiency of care rather than simply seeing more patients. For tech-forward practitioners, "enough" often means reaching the cutting edge of clinical capability.

The Boutique Experience chooses depth over breadth as its expression of "enough." Dr. Tracy Li Cheung's concierge model—12 clinical days per month, over $500,000 in collections per full-time employee—prioritizes intentional, personalized care over volume metrics. The boutique practitioner finds their "enough" in the depth of impact rather than breadth of reach.

The High-Volume Clinic finds "enough" in maximizing accessibility and serving large numbers of families. Dr. Carter Thomas's principle that "everyone deserves excellent care regardless of financial situation" represents success measured by community impact and lives touched. For high-volume practitioners, "enough" might be measured in families served and barriers to care removed.

The Multi-Location Empire can embrace "enough" by building systems that eventually free the founding doctor to focus on bigger purposes. The key is recognizing when the systems are robust enough to operate without constant oversight, freeing them for teaching, mentorship, or philanthropy that leverages their accumulated expertise.

The Lifestyle Practice typically embodies the "enough" principle most clearly. Dr. Brian Rochford's evolution from a $2 million traditional operation to a $5.1 million digital practice working just 27 hours per week demonstrates defining success in terms of freedom and integration rather than just production numbers.

The Startup Journey is actively discovering what "enough" means as values and vision clarify. These practitioners have the advantage of designing their practice intentionally from the beginning, potentially avoiding the expansion trap that catches many successful orthodontists.

The critical insight across all personality types is that "enough" isn't a number—it's an alignment between your practice structure and your life's deeper purpose.

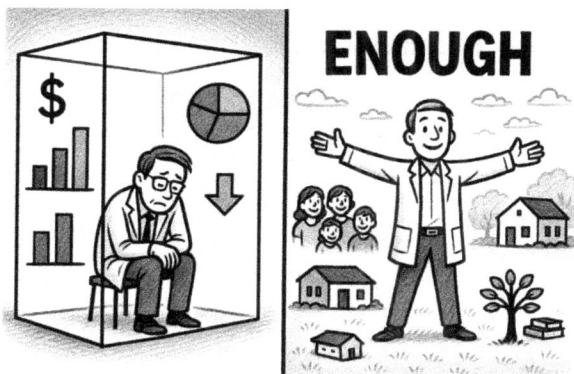

Purpose Beyond Professional Achievement

Here's what I believe, and what guides my approach to both practice and life: **our purpose in life isn't to do great clinical orthodontics or make tons of money and buy three vacation homes. Life and our purpose—it's bigger than that.**

For me, as a Christian, that bigger purpose is to glorify God and serve His creation. This doesn't diminish the importance of clinical excellence—it elevates it by connecting it to something eternal. When I straighten teeth, I'm participating in the work of restoration that reflects God's character.

Your deeper purpose might be different—raising children who change the world, advancing scientific knowledge, building community, creating beauty, serving the marginalized, or pursuing truth in other forms. The specific calling matters less than recognizing that it exists and that it's bigger than your practice.

But here's the beautiful paradox: achieving professional excellence can actually free us to focus on that deeper purpose. A well-run orthodontic practice with proper systems and team development provides the resources and freedom to invest in what truly matters.

The Integration Triangle

This integration of professional excellence and spiritual purpose transforms how you experience your daily work. Think of it as three interconnected gears that must work together harmoniously: **Professional Excellence, Personal Purpose,** and **Spiritual Calling.**

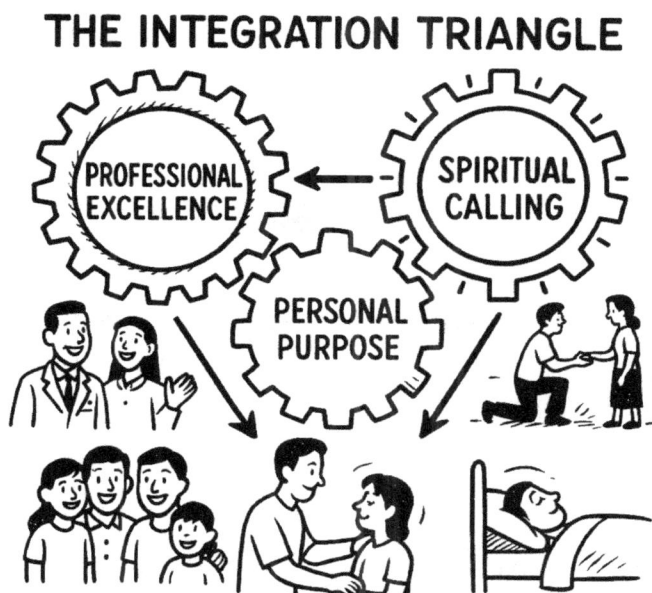

THE INTEGRATION TRIANGLE

When these three dimensions align, they create something powerful. Difficult cases become opportunities to practice perseverance and problem-solving. Challenging team situations become occasions to develop wisdom and compassion. Financial decisions become exercises in stewardship and generosity.

From this central mechanism, the impact radiates outward: exceptional patient care, quality family time, community service, and meaningful relationships all emerge naturally when your practice operates from this integrated foundation.

For those whose worldview differs from mine, the principle remains: **connecting your professional work to something larger than yourself transforms both the work and your experience of doing it.** Whether your larger purpose centers on family legacy, scientific advancement, community service, or philosophical pursuit, the integration creates meaning that transcends the immediate tasks of orthodontic practice.

Getting Off the Hamster Wheel

The hamster wheel of practice life is seductive because it feels productive. You're busy, you're needed, you're making money, you're helping patients. The movement creates an illusion of progress even when you're not actually moving toward anything meaningful.

But busyness isn't the same as purposefulness. Being needed isn't the same as being effective. Making money isn't the same as making a difference.

Getting caught on the hamster wheel helps no one:

- **It doesn't help your patients**, who deserve a practitioner operating from sustainable energy rather than exhaustion

- **It doesn't help your team**, who need inspired leadership rather than reactive management
- **It doesn't help your family**, who need your presence, not just your provision
- **It doesn't help you**, as you miss the very reasons you chose healthcare as a calling

The way off the hamster wheel is to systematize excellence so you can focus your irreplaceable time on irreplaceable activities.

This requires a fundamental shift in thinking from "What else can I do?" to "What can I stop doing?" and "What can someone else do?"

Breaking free from the hamster wheel requires courage to disappoint some people in the short term to serve everyone better in the long term. It means saying no to appointments that don't align with your optimal schedule. It means investing in systems and training that cost money upfront but create freedom later.

HAMSTER WHEEL REALITY

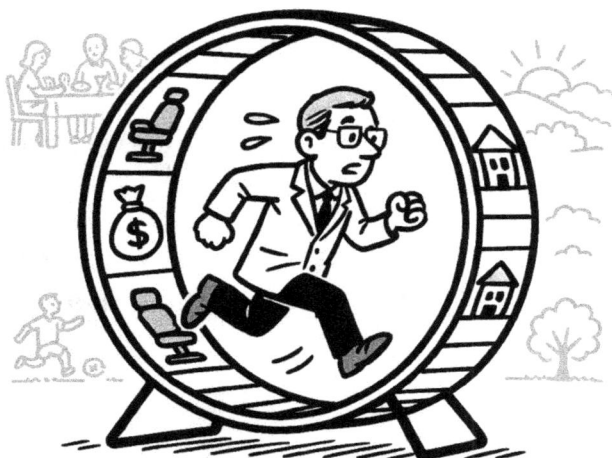

Success Redefined: Your Legacy in the Making

Most orthodontists think about legacy in terms of practice valuation—what they can sell their practice for when they retire. **But true legacy encompasses much more than financial assets.**

Consider what you're actually building beyond the balance sheet:

Time Sovereignty: The ability to control your schedule in ways that align with your priorities. Having every Wednesday afternoon free for family activities, being able to attend your children's school events without stress, or having the flexibility to take extended mission trips.

Quality of Patient Relationships: The depth and satisfaction of the connections you build with patients and families. The orthodontist who treats three generations of the same family has achieved something that no amount of expansion can replicate. **These relationships can't be quantified but often provide more meaning than production metrics.**

Professional Impact: The clinical excellence, innovation, or mentorship that advances the field and lives on after your retirement. Consider the orthodontist who spends their final years systematically documenting their approach to complex cases, creating detailed studies that become invaluable resources for residents and young practitioners. Or the practitioner who develops innovative treatment protocols that colleagues adopt throughout their region, improving patient outcomes long after the originator has retired.

Knowledge Multiplication: The systems, protocols, and innovations you've developed that can benefit others. **The orthodontist who documents their unique approaches, develops training programs for team members, or creates patient education materials has created knowledge assets that multiply their impact.**

Community Investment: The relationships and service that outlast your career. The orthodontist who coaches youth sports for twenty years while running a successful practice leaves a different legacy than the one who postpones all community involvement until after retirement.

[Research shows that healthcare providers who maintain strong patient relationships report 40% higher job satisfaction and 30% lower burnout rates compared to those focused primarily on productivity metrics.]

Your Implementation Path: Making It Real

You don't need to revolutionize your entire practice overnight. **The path to freedom and purpose is paved with small, consistent choices that align your practice with your values rather than external expectations.**

This Month: Define Your "Enough"

Write down specific boundaries that reflect your values:

- What income level would allow you to live comfortably while pursuing your deeper purposes?
- How many patients can you serve excellently without compromising quality or burning out?
- What schedule would give you energy for both exceptional work and meaningful relationships?

This Quarter: Reclaim Your Time

Implement one significant system change:

- Train a team member to handle responsibilities that don't require your unique expertise
- Automate one administrative process that currently consumes your time
- Say no to one commitment that creates obligation without meaningful return

This Year: Align Practice With Purpose

Design your practice to support rather than compete with your life's calling:

- Schedule regular time for family activities that matter to you
- Commit to community service that energizes rather than drains you
- Invest in continuing education that excites rather than obligates you
- Create space for personal development that refreshes your perspective

[Harvard Business Review studies show 80% greater success rates with incremental change versus dramatic transformation attempts.]

The Ultimate Integration

The ultimate practice paradox is this: the better you become at building a practice that doesn't need you for every decision and detail, the more you're freed to do what only you can do.

One seasoned orthodontist discovered this approach after fifteen years of practice. By systematically developing her team and implementing robust systems, she reclaimed significant time each week. Rather than seeing more patients, she chose to mentor young orthodontists, teach advanced techniques at continuing education courses, serve on medical mission trips, and prioritize family commitments.

This shift often leads practitioners to realize they may earn less per hour, but gain more per day—not just financially, but in terms of meaning, impact, and fulfillment. Their practice begins to fund their purpose instead of preventing it.

When your practice serves your purpose rather than consuming it, everything changes:

- **Your professional work becomes more sustainable** because it's connected to something larger than itself
- **Your personal life becomes more fulfilling** because you have the time and energy to invest in what matters most
- **Your deeper calling finds expression** through your work rather than in spite of it

This is the freedom that comes from mastering the practice paradoxes: not freedom from excellence, but freedom for excellence in the areas where you're truly called to make a difference.

The Ripple Effect: Your Legacy in Motion

We all have endless potential, but only when we work through the paradoxes that trap most practitioners in cycles of busyness without purpose. **The impact of one person living with clear purpose and effective systems ripples outward in ways that can't be measured.**

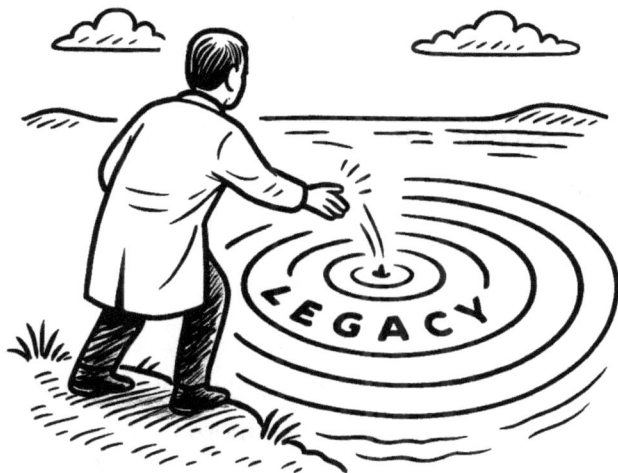

THE RIPPLE EFFECT
OF A LIFE WELL LIVED

Picture yourself as someone planting seeds in rich soil, but instead of plants growing, the seeds sprout into: mentored young doctors, happy families with beautiful smiles, community buildings, knowledge trees with wisdom as leaves, and a strong family tree. Your orthodontic skills, properly stewarded, can fund mission trips, support family priorities, enable community service, or advance scientific knowledge. Your leadership abilities can mentor the next generation of practitioners who will serve thousands of patients you'll never meet.

The most successful orthodontists understand that their highest value is in creating environments where excellent work happens consistently.

Your practice should fund your purpose, not prevent it. When it does, you'll discover that professional success and personal fulfillment are actually complementary forces, not competing priorities, that create a life worth living and a legacy worth leaving.

The choice is yours. The time is now. Your deeper purpose is waiting.

Key Takeaways

- Time is the ultimate currency. You can make more money, but you can't make more time.
- Success without purpose is just busyness in disguise.

- The concept of enough is not about limitation, but about alignment between your practice and your life's purpose.
- Growth for growth's sake builds a treadmill; purpose-driven growth creates freedom and fulfillment.
- Your practice should fund your purpose, not prevent it.

Next Steps

You don't need to overhaul your entire practice overnight to live with purpose. Starting this week, you can:

Define your Enough: Write down what "enough" means for you in income, patient load, and schedule.

Align with Purpose: Choose one action outside of dentistry—family, faith, community—that you will intentionally prioritize this month.

Reflect Weekly: Set aside 15 minutes to reconnect with your "why" and evaluate whether your practice decisions align with it.

We've explored the concept of "enough" and how purpose, rather than endless growth, is the true measure of a life well-lived. When your practice serves your higher calling, success becomes more than numbers on a report; it becomes legacy.

But purpose without action is just potential. All the systems, strategies, and insights in this book lead here: the moment where you decide to live differently. In the next chapter, we'll shift from understanding to implementation and take that higher purpose and put it into practice so your life and work finally align.

Chapter 13: Your Next Steps

By: Dr. Kyle Fagala

Dr. Melissa stared at the stack of sticky notes on her desk. Each one was a reminder of systems she meant to implement months ago. The ideas were good. She knew they'd save time, reduce stress, and give her more freedom. But every day, she got pulled back into the grind of patients, paperwork, and problems. Knowledge wasn't her issue. Action was.

Throughout this book, you've uncovered the hidden paradoxes of orthodontic practice—control, growth, leadership, time, and even success itself. You've learned how to reclaim joy, align your practice with your values, empower your team, protect your health, diversify income, and define what "enough" means. But knowledge alone changes nothing. This final chapter is about bridging that gap and choosing action, committing to change, and creating momentum that carries you forward.

This chapter will guide you in three critical ways:

- Identifying the practice paradox that most directly affects you right now.

- Choosing the first concrete action that will begin resolving it.

- Building a framework to sustain progress without overwhelming yourself.

It's not about doing everything. It's about doing the right next thing

From Insight to Implementation: The Critical Moment

Knowledge without application remains merely potential energy—stored but unused. The principles we've explored throughout this book become powerful only when applied consistently to your unique situation.

This pattern appears repeatedly among orthodontists we've worked with. As one practitioner shared in our research, "I understood everything about efficiency and systems, but I wasn't actually implementing any of it. I kept saying I'd make changes after we reached the next milestone." Her experience illustrates what we see consistently: the breakthrough typically comes when practitioners choose one principle—like training their team as mini-orthodontists—and commit to implementing it completely before moving to the next change.

This is the implementation trap that catches most successful orthodontists: they understand the concepts intellectually but never commit to the messy, uncomfortable work of actually changing how they operate.

Why Smart Orthodontists Struggle with Implementation

Intelligence can be a liability when it comes to change. Smart people are excellent at analyzing problems and understanding solutions. They're also excellent at finding reasons why "now isn't the right time" to implement those solutions.

The orthodontist who can diagnose a tricky Class II malocclusion in seconds often spends months avoiding the obvious changes their practice needs. Why? Because implementation requires temporary discomfort, and intelligent people are skilled at rationalizing why that discomfort should be avoided.

Implementation begins with small, consistent steps rather than dramatic overnight transformations. Think of your practice like steering a ship—changing direction doesn't happen with violent jerking of the wheel, but through subtle, consistent adjustments that gradually alter your course toward your chosen destination.

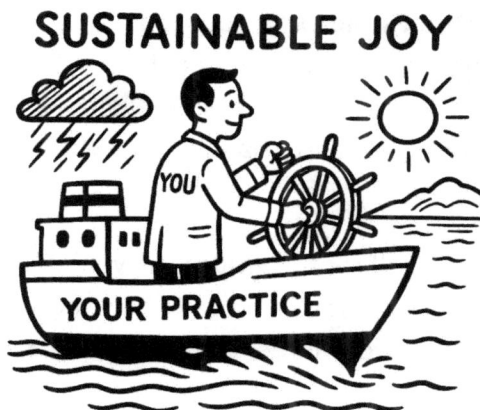

SUSTAINABLE JOY

YOU

YOUR PRACTICE

Your Practice Paradox Diagnostic

Before you can implement solutions, you need clarity on which problem to solve first. **Most orthodontists try to fix everything at once and end up fixing nothing.**

Create a personalized action plan by identifying which practice paradox most directly addresses your current pain point:

The Control Paradox: If you're trapped by the need to personally handle every clinical detail, you're suffocating your practice's potential. Start by training one team member to conduct initial patient evaluations following your protocols. This single change can reclaim 5-10 hours per week.

The Growth Paradox: If you're overwhelmed by trying to serve every type of patient, you're diluting your effectiveness. Clarify your practice personality type and begin attracting your ideal patient population. Say no to patients who don't fit your model.

The Leadership Paradox: If your team depends on you for every decision, you've created a bottleneck that limits everyone's growth. Implement one systematic delegation protocol that empowers your staff to handle routine situations without your input.

The Clinical Excellence Paradox: If you're sacrificing efficiency for perfection, you're actually harming both. Establish clear protocols for your three-wire sequence and IPR procedures that maintain quality while saving time. Perfect is the enemy of excellent.

The Time Paradox: If you never have enough hours in the day, you're managing tasks instead of leading systems. Implement the clinical coordinator role to serve as your practice expeditor and decision-maker for routine issues.

PRACTICE PARADOXES

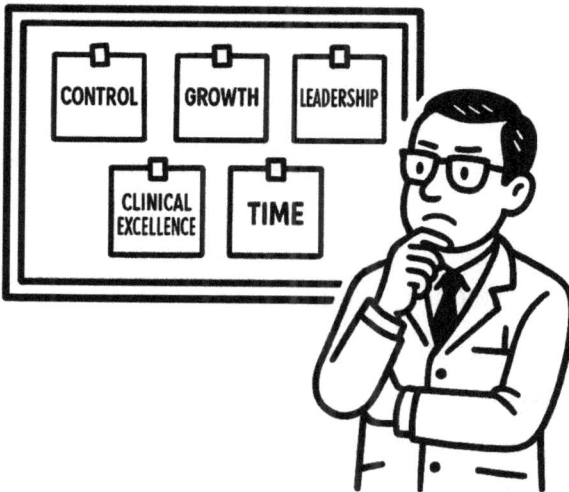

Start with the paradox that creates the most pain in your daily experience. Master one before attempting another.

The 90-Day Sprint: Your Transformation Timeline

Most practice transformation attempts fail because they lack structure and deadlines. **Without a framework, good intentions dissolve into eventual somedays.**

Here's your 90-day sprint to implement one major change:

Days 1-30: Foundation Building

- Choose your primary focus from the five paradoxes above
- Implement one clinical protocol that saves you 15+ minutes daily
- Establish one non-negotiable boundary (family dinner, workout time, no emails after 7 PM)
- Begin training one team member for expanded responsibilities

Week 4 Checkpoint: You should see measurable time savings and feel less reactive to daily interruptions.

Days 31-60: System Development

- **Expand your team member's role** beyond the initial training
- **Create one automated system** that removes you from routine decisions
- **Establish weekly team huddles** with clear agendas and outcomes
- **Document what's working** so you can replicate it

Week 8 Checkpoint: Your team should be handling decisions that previously required your input.

Days 61-90: Integration and Refinement

- Evaluate progress against your initial goals
- Adjust systems based on what you've learned
- Plan your next 90-day sprint for a different paradox
- Celebrate wins and identify areas for continued focus

Week 12 Checkpoint: The change should feel natural, not forced. If it doesn't, you're trying to change too much too fast.

THE 90-DAY SPRINT

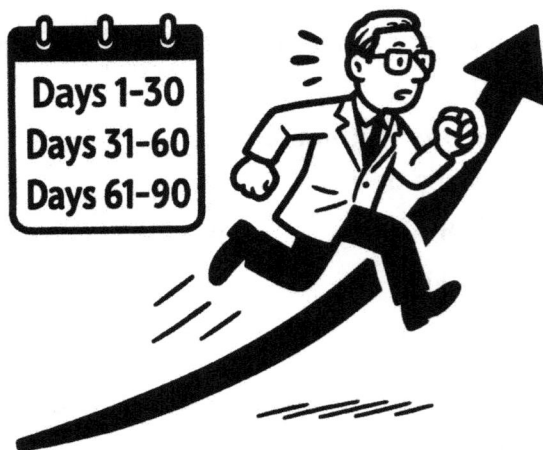

Days 1–30
Days 31–60
Days 61–90

This structured approach prevents overwhelm while building momentum through quick wins that compound into significant transformation.

The Community You Never Knew You Needed

Luke's journey from high-stress entrepreneurship in New York to building purposeful businesses in Pensacola taught him that **isolation amplifies every challenge.**

"When I was trying to figure everything out alone, every setback felt catastrophic," he reflects. "Finding a community of entrepreneurs who understood the balance I was seeking changed everything."

The same principle applies to orthodontic practice. Professional isolation creates blind spots that community can illuminate. When another orthodontist describes their approach to a challenge you've faced, you gain access to possibilities previously invisible to you.

Finding Your Orthodontic Tribe

Look for orthodontists who share your values around practice-life integration rather than just focusing on production metrics. The practitioner committed to working 27 hours per week, like Dr. Brian Rochfor,d will offer different wisdom than the one building a multi-location empire, even though both approaches can be successful.

Digital communities have eliminated geographic barriers. Virtual masterminds, orthodontic Facebook groups focused on lifestyle practices, and online forums connect practitioners across continents. The key lies in active participation—asking thoughtful questions and sharing genuine insights rather than passive consumption.

Consider starting small. Perhaps connect with just two or three orthodontists facing similar challenges. These intimate relationships often prove more valuable than large professional networks because they allow for the vulnerability necessary for real growth.

My experience building Saddle Creek Orthodontics while raising a family required finding mentors who had successfully
navigated similar terrain. The orthodontists who inspired me
most weren't necessarily the highest producers. They were
the ones who had figured out how to excel professionally
while being present for their families.

Resources That Actually Matter

**Your development as a balanced orthodontist requires
ongoing learning, but not all learning is created equal.**
Focus on resources that address the integration of clinical excellence with personal fulfillment rather than just technical or
business knowledge.

High-Impact Learning

Books: Look beyond purely dental texts to include leadership,
systems thinking, and life integration resources. Stephen Cov-
ey's *7 Habits of Highly Effective People* remains foundational
for understanding how professional choices should align with
personal values.

Podcasts: Find shows hosted by healthcare professionals
who've successfully integrated their practices with their life
priorities. The insights from these conversations often prove
more valuable than generic business advice.

Continuing Education: Choose courses that address practice systems and team development, not just clinical techniques. **The orthodontist who masters delegation and team leadership often achieves better outcomes than the one who only pursues the latest clinical innovations.**

Practice Management Consultants: Work with advisors who understand that efficiency should create freedom, not just higher production. The right consultant helps you build systems that serve your chosen practice persona rather than pushing you toward a one-size-fits-all growth model.

Peer Groups: Join or form small groups of orthodontists committed to practice-life integration. These relationships provide accountability, perspective, and encouragement during the inevitable challenges of practice transformation.

Measuring What Actually Matters

The ultimate measure of your practice's success isn't found in monthly production reports or patient volume but in your sustained experience of meaningful joy.

This metric transcends conventional success markers, though it often correlates with them. Many practitioners discover this distinction when they realize their highest production months often coincide with their lowest life satisfaction.

The pattern is common: celebrating financial milestones while personal relationships suffer, or achieving professional recognition while sacrificing health and family time. The breakthrough often comes when success gets redefined to include meaningful relationships, personal energy, and genuine satisfaction with professional choices.

Quarterly Assessment Questions

Set reminders to regularly evaluate not just conventional metrics but experiential ones:

- **Energy Check:** Does your work energize or deplete you?
- **Relationship Quality:** Do patient interactions feel meaningful or rushed?
- **Priority Alignment:** Does your schedule reflect your stated priorities?
- **Presence Test:** Are you present for the family moments that matter most?
- **Growth Gauge:** Are you growing as a clinician and as a person?

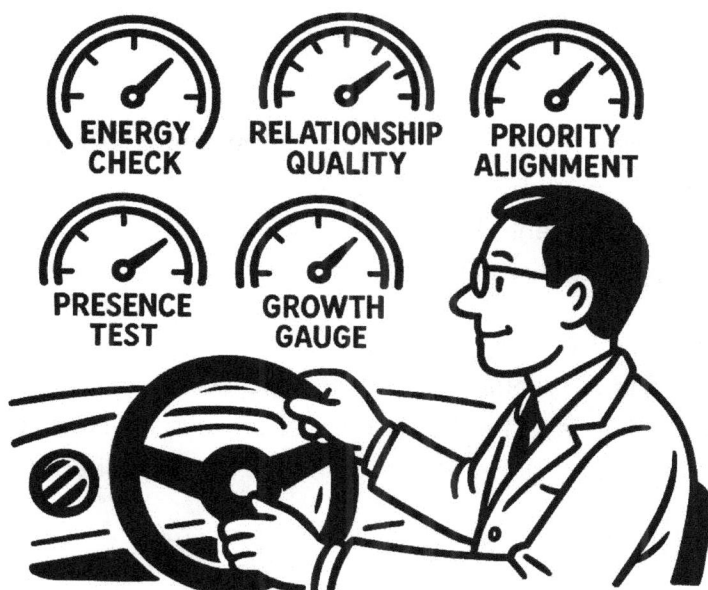

THE JOY DASHBOARD

These questions reveal alignment gaps that require attention before they become major problems.

The Implementation Mindset: Progress Over Perfection

Remember that implementation is more about progress than perfection. Every orthodontic practice encounters seasons of misalignment and drift. The distinguishing factor between thriving and struggling practices isn't the absence of challenges but the response to them.

Luke learned this lesson while building multiple businesses. "The companies that survived were the ones that had systems for recognizing problems early and processes for addressing them quickly."

View setbacks as information rather than failure. Each challenge provides data about what's working and what needs adjustment. This perspective allows for constructive refinement rather than discouragement.

Kyle's journey building Saddle Creek Orthodontics alongside a growing family required constant application and refinement of these principles. "The balance I seek is a dynamic equilibrium that requires ongoing attention as life's seasons change."

The Continuous Refinement Cycle

Professional development works most effectively as a continuous cycle rather than a linear progression:

1. **Implement** one system or change
2. **Assess** the results after 30-60 days
3. **Adjust** based on what you've learned
4. **Expand** to the next area needing attention

This virtuous cycle creates momentum that transforms isolated improvements into comprehensive practice transformation.

THE FIRST STEP

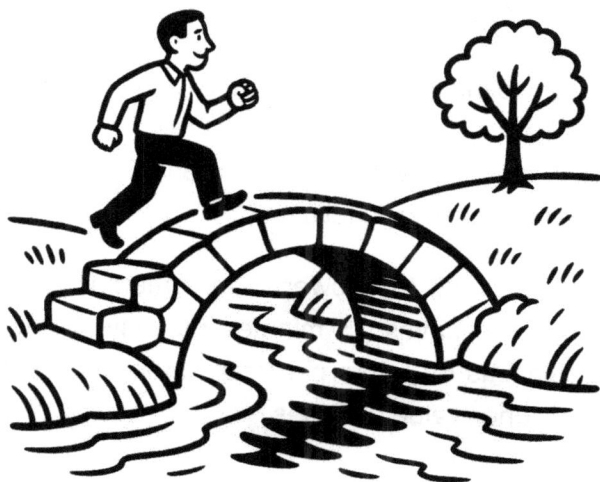

As you begin implementing these principles, remember that the practice paradox is resolved by reimagining what success looks like altogether. Start where you are.

When faced with decisions, ask yourself: **"Am I choosing momentary relief at the expense of lasting fulfillment?"** The practices that seem most demanding in the moment—implementing new systems, establishing boundaries, delegating responsibility—often yield the greatest long-term joy.

The Compound Effect of Small Changes

Small steps compound into transformation. The wire sequence you simplify today will save you time for months. The team member you train this week will handle responsibilities for years to come. The boundary you establish now protects what matters most indefinitely.

Don't underestimate the power of incremental change. The orthodontist who saves 15 minutes per day through better systems reclaims 65 hours per year—more than a full work week—for higher-value activities.

Key Takeaways

- Insight without action is wasted potential. The turning point comes when you implement.
- You don't have to fix everything at once. Start with the paradox causing the most pain.
- Small, consistent changes compound into transformative results.
- Your practice should enhance your life, not consume it. Implementation is how that happens.

Next Steps

You don't need a complete overhaul. Start where you are:

Identify one paradox – Control, Growth, Leadership, Clinical Excellence, or Time. Which one limits you most right now?

Choose one change – Delegate a routine responsibility, set a boundary, simplify a protocol, or train a team member.

Commit for 90 days – Focus on this single change until it becomes part of your normal rhythm.

Build accountability – Share your commitment with a peer, mentor, or team member who will help you stay on track.

The Practice of Your Dreams

With the principles you've learned, the orthodontic practice of your dreams is inevitable. But it won't happen by accident. It requires the same intentionality you bring to complex clinical cases. It demands the same systematic thinking you apply to treatment planning. It needs the same persistent refinement you give to your clinical skills.

The difference is that this time, you're not just improving your technique—you're designing your life.

Trust the process. Embrace the paradox. And watch as both your practice and your life transform.

Conclusion

Sunday evenings are different for Dr. James, now that he's addressed the practice paradox. The quiet joy and anticipation he feels are a far cry from the dread that once knotted his stomach. Now, as he sits at the table with his family, he is present. He laughs with his kids and listens, really listens to their stories, and feels eager about the week ahead. His wife catches his eye across the table, but this time it's not a glance of weariness. It's a smile, a quiet acknowledgment that he is here with them, fully. The table is filled with conversation, laughter, and the warmth of a family connected. Monday morning no longer looms as a threat; it feels like an opportunity. He gets to fulfill his mission, lead his team with clarity, and continue building the life he once only dreamed of.

Throughout this book, we've named the paradox at the heart of so many practices: outward success that masks inner exhaustion. We've seen how the very traits that help build thriving offices, discipline, drive, and perfectionism can also drain the joy out of the work. We've walked through the hidden costs of unchecked growth, micromanagement, disconnection, and the relentless pursuit of "more."

But we've also seen that another way is possible. By examining the paradoxes of control, leadership, growth, and time, we've uncovered what it takes to create not just a prosperous practice, but a fulfilling life. The journey is not about sacrifice; it's about integration. The practice should serve your life, not consume it.

Through the six domains we've explored–Fulfillment, Communication, Leadership, Growth, Life Beyond the Clinic, and Purpose–you now hold a blueprint for real transformation. These are not abstract ideas. They are practical tools: the JOY framework, the Practice Paradox Diagnostic, and the 90-Day Sprint. They are habits and systems designed to bring you back to what matters most: joy in your work, clarity in your purpose, and alignment between your practice and your life.

The choice now is yours. Will you continue down the same road, successful on paper but hollow inside, or will you take the courageous step to redefine success on your own terms? Purpose without action is only potential. Change begins when you choose one paradox to address, one action to take, one step forward into the life you've been waiting for.

We've witnessed this transformation firsthand. Doctors who once rarely made it home in time for dinner or missed their kids' recitals, games, and school events now make it a point to be there. They sit down at the table, share meals with their families, cheer from the sidelines, and spend unhurried time with their spouses. They are no longer spectators in their own lives, but active participants in the relationships that matter most. Practices once sustained by sheer willpower now thrive because they are built on systems, clarity, and purpose. The orthodontist you were meant to be, clinically excellent, personally fulfilled, and purposefully integrated, is within reach.

The good life is not found in accumulating more. It is found in cultivating enough. Enough success to feel fulfilled, enough systems to be free, enough purpose to stay driven, and enough wisdom to remain balanced.

Your paradox ends here. The roadmap is in your hands. The rest is up to you.

Epilogue: Your Journey Beyond the Practice Paradox

You came to this book because something felt wrong. You can change this.

Imagine walking out of your office on a clear afternoon, the sun still high, and heading straight to your child's game or to meet a loved one. Imagine leading a team that thrives without your constant oversight, freeing you to focus on the moments and relationships that matter most. Imagine looking ahead to the week not with dread, but with gratitude because your work is aligned with who you are and the life you want to live.

This is the promise of living beyond the paradox. It isn't about perfection. It isn't about eliminating every challenge or obstacle. It's about integration, bringing your values, your purpose, and your practice into harmony so that they fuel, rather than fight, each other.

We've seen it happen: doctors who once felt trapped by their success now speak with clarity and live with joy. Teams once fractured by stress now move with unity. Families once strained by absence now feel whole again. These aren't abstract dreams; they are real transformations made possible by choosing a different path.

The future is not waiting for you somewhere far off. It begins here, in the next decision you make. To live with balance. To practice with joy. To lead with purpose. To love with presence.

The paradox is no longer your story. The new story is yours to write, one that begins not with burnout, but with freedom, fulfillment, and the quiet confidence of a life well lived.

"The good life is built, not on the accumulation of more, but on the cultivation of enough—enough success to be fulfilled, enough systems to be free, enough purpose to be driven, and enough wisdom to know when these elements have found their proper balance."

— Dr. Kyle Fagala & Luke Infinger

About the Authors

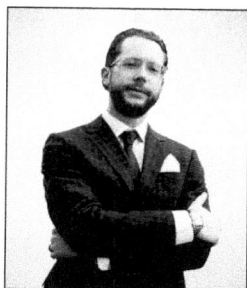

Luke Infinger is the Founder and CEO of HIP, a leading growth agency serving orthodontists, dentists, and healthcare professionals nationwide. A serial entrepreneur and business strategist, Luke has helped hundreds of practices accelerate patient growth, streamline operations, and build sustainable, purpose-driven businesses. After earning his degree from SCAD and working in New York, he returned to his hometown of Pensacola, Florida, where he launched HIP from a small apartment. Over the past decade, he has scaled the agency to over 8-figures by focusing on systems, not just inspiration. Today, Luke also co-leads Ion Growth Agency with Dr. Kyle Fagala, while living on a farm outside Pensacola with his wife Kathryn and their two children, Aislinn and Ezra.

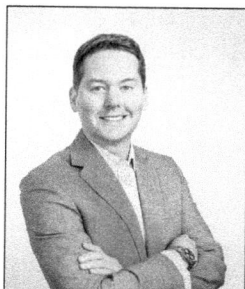

Dr. Kyle Fagala is the owner of Saddle Creek Orthodontics in Memphis and co-founder of Neon Canvas, a digital marketing agency. A trusted authority and sought-after speaker, he helps orthodontists grow practices with strategies grounded in real-world experience. He hosts The Digital Orthodontist: Live! podcast, authored two children's books—All The Best Faces Wear Braces and There's Nothing Finer Than Aligners— and serves as a Key Opinion Leader for 3M Oral Care. Dr. Kyle teaches Development of Occlusion at the University of Tennessee Health Science Center and lives in Germantown with his wife Anna, their four children, and an Aussiedoodle named Sammie.